THE DOWNGRADING OF AMERICAN HEALTHCARE

How Regulatory and Cultural Forces Continue to Negatively Impact the Healthcare System in the United States

Camilo R. Gomez, M.D., M.B.A.
Neurological Institute of Alabama
Birmingham, Alabama

THIS IS A CREATESPACE BOOK
Published by On-Demand Publishing, LLC

CreateSpace
7290 B. Investment Drive
Charleston, SC 29418
USA

www.createspace.com
www.amazon.com

Library of Congress Cataloging-in-Publication Data

Gomez, Camilo R.
The Downgrading of American Healthcare. How Regulatory and Cultural Forces Continue to Negatively Impact The Healthcare System in the United States / Camilo R. Gomez – 1st Ed

p. cm.

ISBN-13: 978-1475069822
ISBN-10: 1475069820

I. American Healthcare. II. Camilo R. Gomez

LCCN: 2012915734

Manufactured in the United States of America

Dedication

To my children, Cristina and Camilo, my most important legacy to our Country

ACKNOWLEGMENTS

This book would not have been possible without the counsel, assistance and encouragement of many individuals along the way, and I would like to take a moment to acknowledge them. To begin, the people at Create Space afforded me the opportunity and means to bring the book to publication with phenomenal ease, while its parent company Amazon provided the marketing and sales expertise necessary to disseminate it. Although I personally authored the majority of the illustrations, the basic art I used (i.e. stick figures) is by Daniel Tero from Leap In, Ltd (United Kingdom), and was made available through www.iStockphoto.com.

I am very grateful to the various colleagues, all kindred spirits, with whom I have enjoyed innumerable discussions about the state of our country and our profession, particularly Cole A. Giller, Constantine Athanasuleas, James D. Geyer, Hector Caballero, Diane Counce, Bradley Cavender, Gordon J. Kirshberg, J. Christopher Davis, and Michael D. McKinney. They have all served as a sounding board for the opinions I express in the book and contributed to its realization by virtue of their perspective. My gratitude extends to my nurse practitioner, Wendy W. Conner, one of the best partners I have ever had; who has endured on a daily basis my litany of complaints about the hurdles we encounter in our daily practice.

Moreover, she was also exceedingly helpful during the review and copyediting of the chapters that address issues in nursing. I would also like to acknowledge Dr. Christine Agee, who, after listening to me for what seemed like innumerable hours, independently and concurrently came to the conclusion that I should seriously consider putting my thoughts and energy into writing a book; one that would address my concerns about the topics we had been discussing; well, here it is!

I want to recognize the men for whom I have worked over the years; Simon Horenstein, my mentor and first program director, who introduced me to the virtues of the Socratic method of education, to the rewards of applying critical thinking to medical situations, and to the benefits of insightful skepticism regarding scientific publications. Next, John B. Selhorst, my first chairman as a faculty member in St. Louis University; who believed in my ability to develop and execute his vision of an academic stroke center at a time when such an idea was still embryonic; he provided me with the opportunity to create the *Souers Stroke Institute*, and to direct it until 1995. Finally, the late John N. Whitaker, my chairman during my last tenure as part of the *medical intelligentsia* at the University of Alabama at Birmingham (UAB). His strength, vision and determination helped me build a unique clinical entity; a model for comprehensive stroke centers that, at its zenith, was arguably the first cradle for the pioneering adepts in Interventional Neurology.

Along these lines, it is fitting for me to mention the graduates from our UAB Fellowship Program; those courageous souls who entered into the battle zone we created to forge the specialists in our field; those that endured the vicissitudes of a grueling program not made for the faint of heart; the ones that survived and completed the program; my academic children: Morgan S Campbell, Sean C. Orr, Rodney D. Soto, Ali R. Malek, Susana M. Bowling, Srinath Kadimi and Pramod Sethi. They taught me as much as I taught them, and I am very proud of their accomplishments and success!

On a more pragmatic note, I could not have completed the passages on compensation and billing without the assistance of James E. Stidham and his team, particularly Jackie Bailey. Over the last five years, Jim has turned out to be a phenomenal business partner and has done more for me that I will ever be able to repay him. He was also kind enough to help during the review of a number of other chapters dealing with regulatory issues. Likewise, Sheila O. McKenna provided me with important information and statistics on physician compensation; both Sue Esleck and Camille Filoromo shared inside information relative to the national changes on quality indicators and core measures. I am indebted to all three of them for their assistance.

Finally, I have the deepest appreciation for Elizabeth G. Gonzalez and Kayla K. Fricks. Their editorial commentaries during the copyediting process proved to be very insightful and balanced.

Camilo R. Gomez

An Initial Thought...

He who knows not and knows not that he knows not is a fool...

...Shun him!

He who knows not and knows that he knows not is a child...

...Teach him!

He who knows and knows not that he knows is asleep...

...Wake him!

He who knows and knows that he knows is wise...

...Follow him!

Old Chinese Proverb

Table of Contents

INTRODUCTION **13**

FUNDAMENTAL DOWNGRADING

1. Principles of Medical Practice 27
2. Evidence Based Medicine 40
3. Problem Oriented Medical Diagnosis 55
4. Medical Education 68
5. Nursing Education 92

PRACTICAL DOWNGRADING

6. Polypharmacy & Psychopathology 107
7. Physician Compensation 123
8. Regulation of Conflicts of Interest 141
9. Medical Malpractice 157
10. Allied Health Professions 173

HOSPITAL DOWNGRADING

11. The Joint Commission 191
12. Nursing Leadership 205
13. Physician Leadership 219
14. Quality and Safety Measures 232
15. Hospital Protocols & Policies 252
16. Emergencies 274
17. Pain 284

CULTURAL AND REGULATORY DOWNGRADING

18. Entitlements 301
19. Patient Education 315

20. Treatment Complications 328
21. Generic Medications 340
22. Paperwork 356
23. Patient Privacy 372

Final Remarks & Outlook 389

SELECTED READING 413

INTRODUCTION

On Friday, August 5th, 2011, the rating agency of Standard and Poor downgraded the national credit of the United States to AA+ from AAA, where it had been since 1917.[1] This unprecedented action resulted from the inability of the present administration to demonstrate a reasonable and effective plan for the long-term management of the national debt. This attitude was neither new nor surprising, since the government of the United States (both Republican and Democrat) for many years has failed to balance national budgets, reduce spending of federal funds, and contain the ever-increasing debt, which, as of this writing, surpasses $16 trillion. Although at the national level this credit downgrade triggered a major debate of whether it was justified or fair, many (including myself) were of the opinion that it should not have been surprising for a country to lose its stellar credit rating when all the government officials could propose was to continue to spend like drunken sailors. After all, would it not be expected for any private citizen's credit score to be reduced should he fail to pay his bills? And, would it not be impossible for such an individual to obtain additional

---

[1] As this book goes to print, the U.S. credit rating was once again downgraded by the rating firm of Egan-Jones from AAA to AA-

credit if he were to keep such a negative balance of revenues and expenditures?

It occurred to me, following such an event, that if there existed a rating agency responsible for scoring healthcare as if it were credit, a similar downgrading of the American healthcare should have already taken place. How so? Well, as someone who has been practicing medicine in the United States for over three decades, I have been a front seat witness of changes that have been forced on all of us primarily due to regulatory processes and government intervention. These two have negatively influenced what is perhaps the most important service industry in our society, both directly as well as indirectly by triggering a whole set of cultural changes that are palpable in every day interactions between physicians and patients. In fact, it seemed more than reasonable that, if an incompetent financial behavior on the part of our government resulted in the nation's credit being downgraded, similarly dysfunctional behavior could have certainly led to detrimental changes in the fundamental core of American medicine, resulting in its downgrade by any reasonable standard. To put it in other words, in looking around our current environment, it is possible to paraphrase former President Ronald Reagan, as we are definitely no longer a *"shiny clinic on the hill"*.

The unhappiness, frustration and cynicism that the changes alluded to have created among physicians who have been practicing medicine for many years are widespread. In fact, not one day goes by that I do not find myself discussing with my colleagues any one of the topics that I will describe in this book. Furthermore, for years now, I (as well as others) have openly expressed relevant opinions regarding these subjects despite the fact that no one seems to be listening. We have been particularly vocal every time surprising changes are imposed on our daily activities in order to fulfill some government mandate, regardless of whether it benefits patients or not. At the time of this writing, this seems to occur on a weekly basis, making every Monday the source of depressing expectations. Unfortunately, having a dissenting opinion about the state of affairs when one is not in control of how the system operates can conveniently lead to one being labeled as a "Disruptive Physician", with all the consequences attached to such an appellative and being tantamount to clinical suicide. And here lies the core motivation for this book: An *exposé* of the most salient regulatory and cultural changes that currently create an increasingly negative climate for the practice of medicine; an insider's view of different issues that are not commonly part of the public debate or the political discourse; an account of how filled with unintended consequences the decisions made by politicians and bureaucrats are when it comes to the outcome of patients. My point of view is simple, and I hope to make a case for it: *It is the progressive government intervention into what we now call healthcare that should be considered the root cause of the bulk of the problems we face!* Just as the entire country has been the target of a progressive government agenda for the last 100 years, so has been medical care as a subset of our societal issues. Furthermore, it is the continued expansion and overreach of government into medical care that has brought us to the present situation and, unless we expose it, discuss it, and analyze it, we will not have a prayer of a chance of fixing it. Moreover, additional government involvement is certainly destined to sink us!

The book is divided into sections, each one with several chapters. The first section deals with the downgrading process as it affects the fundamental values of sound medical practice. I begin by setting the philosophical conflict between how medicine was intended to operate, and how it has been transformed by the introduction of important changes in thinking and education strategies. It should be easy to see the hand of the government in all these changes, as well as the impact it has had on changing the intellectual culture of American medicine. In the second section, I cover more practical problems. Those that essentially interfere with the day-to-day delivery of care by imposing hurdles and making the system more inefficient than it should be. Some of these, as we will see, directly evolve from some of the ones covered in the first section. Others address the commoditization of medicine, the class warfare waged against physicians, and the unfair ethical discrimination we have been subjected by people whose ethics are at best questionable. The third section speaks to issues relative to hospital operations. I cannot overemphasize its importance since hospitals are organizations that operate completely out of the control of practicing physicians, and yet we depend so much on their performance to be able to deliver certain aspects of medical care. The section addresses deficiencies in hospital leadership structures and their reasons, analyzes the irrational practices they implement, and exposes the most blatant examples of government regulatory control of their activities, always with the excuse of *"looking after the public interest"*. Finally, in the last section, I discuss various cultural changes that are noticeable in the our patients and their families; changes resulting from either their reaction to stimuli created by the healthcare system itself, or as extensions to societal behaviors that are generally apparent in other aspects of everyday life. Additionally, this section exposes some regulatory downgrading that impacts the relationship we have with patients. I organized the book in such a way as to convey a sense of logical structure, although the reader should quickly realize that the topics are so interlaced, that I constantly cross-reference the chapters with each other. I also have to clarify that, even though I have never recorded the conversations I use as examples in the book, all anecdotes are real and taken from my daily experiences. I have used them to emphasize points that may seem on the surface to be incredible. Believe me, you can't make this stuff up!

It is only fair that I explain who I am, as well as how my personal and professional experiences have shaped my perspective; particularly because I am certain that some of the passages in the book are liable to engender controversy. I was born in a small town in the eastern part of the island of Cuba. Following the ascent to power of Fidel Castro in 1959, the situation in that country became untenable for the majority of business owners, including my father. Therefore, as many others did, we emigrated in the mid-1960s and eventually reached Venezuela, the country where I grew up. According to my family, I expressed my inclination to become a physician at a very early age, and continued to nurture such a desire until eventually I was able to fulfill my dream. Due to the progressive decline of the political environment in Venezuela, it became more practical for me to go to medical school in the Dominican Republic. Therefore, at the young age of 16, I left the house of my parents and embarked on an adventure that has become the center of most of my life.

By the time I graduated from medical school, the political situation in Venezuela was so bad [2], that it seemed impractical for me to return to that country to practice

---

[2] President Luis Herrera Campins was in power, leading a succession of heads of state that created the perfect storm from which current president Hugo Chavez originated.

medicine. This circumstance, combined with the fact that most of my classmates were American citizens and regularly advised me of the benefits of postgraduate education in the United States, made my decision to immigrate to our country a very easy one. I completed my neurology postgraduate education in St. Louis University Medical Center, and remained there as a member of its faculty for a total of thirteen years. During this period, I joined the U.S. Army Reserve as a medical officer; this afforded me the opportunity to be in active duty during the Gulf War in 1991. The University of Alabama in Birmingham recruited me sometime later, and I remained in that institution for a total of eight years. Following the tragic accidental death of my boss, the political climate of the University became such that I had no choice but to leave, and I have been in private practice for the last nine years. So, all in all, I spent a total of 23 years as part of the academic community, or what I will recurrently refer to as the *medical intelligentsia*, a fact I want the reader to keep in mind whenever I express a critical view of it.

It is also worth mentioning that, traditionally, neurology has been a specialty that has attracted very intellectual but not very aggressive type of individuals. In fact, an unconfirmed reference to the notable Houston Cardiovascular Surgeon Denton Cooley relates how years ago he summed up a commonly held opinion about neurologists in one statement: *"Neurologists don't treat diseases, they admire them!"* This perception has been detrimental to those of us who thought neurology was a clinical field ripe for evolution into more therapeutic endeavors. In fact, my experience and neurologic practice have been completely opposite to such opinion. To begin, my first year of postgraduate education (i.e. internship) included nine months rotating through intensive care units. During the three years that followed (i.e. residency) I was always primarily responsible for the care of neurologic patients that needed intensive care. Once my postgraduate education was completed, I dedicated the bulk of my practice, research and teaching to the field of cerebrovascular diseases (i.e. stroke). Then, around 1993, not content with spending most of my time dealing with very ill stroke patients or patients that required neurological intensive care, I decided to expand my horizon by venturing into the field of neurointervention. To expand on this for the reader that is not conversant with this concept, it is similar to the evolution of cardiology, which culminated in the development of interventional cardiology (i.e. the treatment of coronary insufficiency by placement of stents and such). Mind you that, in 1993, there were essentially almost no interventional neurologists and it took several of us many years to get to the point where it is now a widely accepted subspecialty, with practitioners everywhere in the world. At the time of this writing, I have been practicing neurology for approximately 32 years and I have been performing neurologic interventions for almost 20 years. In fact, I have spent most of my professional life inside intensive care units and catheterization laboratories. The reader should be astute enough to deduce that my personality is not one to just "admire diseases". In fact, more than one person has said that I am opinionated, arrogant, overbearing and a difficult debate opponent. I concede that such a view may be at least partially accurate. That said, I make no apologies, and in the words of Popeye the Sailor: *"I 'yams what I am, and dats all that I 'yams!"*

I submit, however, that there is more to me than those harsh appellatives. The inquisitive researcher, the Socratic educator, and the critical thinker all live within my worn out body as roommates and partners that together address the various responsibilities of their host. I have very strong views on education and quality, as I believe we should never stop learning and we should strive to achieve excellence in anything we do. This makes me considerably demanding within a society that strives on mediocrity. In my defense, I have never asked any one of my subordinates to carry out an activity that I was not prepared to do myself, arguably better and faster. As an example of this *mélange* of attributes, when I was in my mid-40s, I went back to school and earned a Master of Business Administration degree from the University of Tennessee in Knoxville. That was in fact my first deliberate attempt at understanding some of the problems I outline in the following chapters. It was a first step towards communicating in a professional environment bogged down with regulatory mandates, pseudoscientific rhetoric, and handicapped priorities. Learning about business sparked a personal interest in national economics, finance, and overall policy. Curiously, I discovered this late in my life a strong conservative political tendency, and an obsessive admiration for free markets and the Austrian school of economics. Along these lines, just like Milton Friedman and Charles Murray, I consider myself a lowercase libertarian who abhors government intervention in our daily lives, especially medical practice. I admire Ayn Rand and her work, and I find the objectivist philosophy to suit me just fine. To the critics of Objectivism and their notion that it is just egoism and lack of concern for others, I offer what I call *"The Yellow Mask Philosophy of Life"*. It goes like this: The next time you are sitting in a commercial airliner, and you are being lectured on safety issues, pay attention to what you are told: *"When the yellow masks drop from the ceiling, put yours on first; BEFORE you try to help anyone else!"* Therefore, in everyday life, I submit that we are incapable of truly helping anyone unless we have taken care of ourselves first.

I ask the reader to take everything I have said into account in order to gain insight into the perspective from which I write. I am sure there will be disagreements about my position regarding various topics and I do not mind this. My main interest is to bring to light aspects about our healthcare system that are not commonly heard during the political discourse, from either the left or the right, and which have transformed my profession to a state that is deplorable but the details of which are not very publicly discussed. For example, in a recent episode of the television show *Stossel*, a young physician took the specious position of defending the Affordable Care Act. She kept repeating a popular phrase spewed as a justification for many ill-conceived ideas: *"Our healthcare system is broken!"* However, I suspect that if she had been asked (and for that matter if anyone making the same statement were ever asked) to enumerate the different aspects of the system that are "broken", she would not have been able to come up with a cohesive answer. Well, here it is! I want the following pages to become a good start for anyone who wishes to get an idea of the things that are wrong with our medical system. Bear in mind that I am also of the opinion that, at least when I first came to our country, there still was a great degree of what I have come to call the *American Medical Exceptionalism.* Just as the United States represents a unique republic among all other nations, medicine in our country used to have no parallel; and do not let anyone tell you otherwise! Any one of us, who have sampled how medicine is practiced in other countries, including European nations, can vouch for such a difference; as can any foreign citizen that has sought specialized medical care by traveling to one of many institutions in the United States. Whether any of our Medical Exceptionalism remains today is, at best, debatable.

One additional point I must make is my disdain for the term "Healthcare". I favor the opinion that "health" does not need to be cared for, and that the introduction of this term to replace "Medical Care" underscores how so many non-physician groups want to wedge themselves as stakeholders and drivers of the system. Make no mistake; the orgy of political correctness that currently sweeps our nation takes no exception for medicine. As such, there is the notion that, by changing how we label certain aspects of our lives, we can alter their fundamental fabric with impunity. This type of behavior has been best illustrated by the late humorist George Carlin who referred to the people who promote such changes as the "Human Fulfillment Movement" (i.e. the people who transformed "toilet paper" into "bathroom tissue"), emphasizing their "feel good" and "touchy feely" nomenclature, and little substantive meaning. Thus, at least in my view, the more appropriate term "Medical Care", traditionally used to designate the relationship between a patient and his physician (and everything secondary to that), did not need to be replaced for another that appeared more palatable to all the ancillary individuals that have wanted a "piece of the action". I also contend that it is *precisely* the change from "medical care" to "healthcare" that marked the beginning of the downgrading process, as well as all of its well known consequences, particularly inflated cost and lower quality, the two variables that determine value. In this context, I admit that I struggled when choosing the title of the book until I finally realized that it is precisely this new form of system, the one we call "Healthcare", that which is downgraded anyway. At that moment, it seemed fitting to apply it to the book title without hesitation or remorse. Later, it occurred to me that there was another practical aspect to choosing this term instead of the old traditional one: It may entice more people into reading this book since they may relate to the newer term better because of their familiarity with it. As I expose my position on the various topics covered in this book, the distinction that I have made between these two terms will become evident to the reader, as will my reasons for thinking the way I do.

A few structural and stylistic points also deserve mention. First, some may consider that several of the chapters have an excessive number of illustrations, making the book look like a didactic tome. However, I am a very visual person and, after being an educator for so long, it is at times difficult not to come across overly scholastic. Second, you will find the term "clinical" used many times throughout the book. In case you are a layperson, let me just say that this is a time-honored appellative, derived from the Greek *klinikos* and the Latin *clinicus*, meaning, "To recline in bed". It refers to any person or activity working at the bedside of patients. I use this term emphatically to differentiate anything that directly relates to the practice of medicine from anything that belongs within the realm of bureaucracy. I want the reader to understand the differences between what is thought or planned at administrative levels, and what really happens during patient care. Third, I wish no individual or institution to feel singled out by my remarks. I have made every effort to avoid unfair discrimination by treating all groups within the healthcare environment in the most general way I could. Moreover, the fact that the examples and some illustrations concern my local reality is simply a matter of practicality rather than finger pointing. I think all of us have some degree of responsibility in the problems being discussed, a point that I will cover further in the last chapter in which I explore potential solutions. Fourth, the book is written in first person because it represents my own personal views. I generally have attempted to use the singular form for my exposition, reserving the plural to include common tasks shared by the physician community in general, or to implicitly invite the reader to ponder about a specific concept or controversy. I am not sure that this distinction is uniform throughout the book, but during the editing process, I have kept whichever form seemed better suited to the context in which it was being used. Along the same lines, I have alternatively addressed you, the reader, in either the second or third person, depending upon how intimate I want my remarks to be at that particular point. I beg your indulgence for this stylistic license I have allowed myself. Finally, my use of the third person singular pronouns follows the recommendation made by Charles Murray, which I have found sensible and practical: To assign that of the gender of the senior author, in this case *he*.

It is my hope that, after all is said and done, the reader finds these pages enlightening and that the passages in them lead to introspection, reflection, and circumspection. At a time when I begin to look at the sunset of my medical career, I could have thought of nothing better than to leave behind some type of summary of what many of us think needs attention in our medical system. I pray that this book will fulfill such a niche.

Camilo R. Gomez, MD, MBA
Birmingham, Alabama
Summer of 2012

FUNDAMENTAL DOWNGRADING

1

Principles of Medical Practice

"Reverence for life affords me my fundamental principle of morality"

Albert Schweitzer
French Physician, Philosopher & Missionary
(1875 - 1965)

In order to properly place in perspective the changes that have occurred in American healthcare over the last 40 or 50 years, and which I submit have contributed to its downgrading, we must first review the fundamental principles of medical practice. Those that most of us thought were to guide our professional careers when we originally decided to dedicate our lives to the healing of the sick. Personally, I have always thought the entire realm of medicine was based on a fundamental contract between a patient and his physician. After all, through the ages, the Hippocratic Oath was largely considered a binding agreement the physician would embrace for the benefit of his patients. As such, just as it is with marriage, this basic relationship inherently requires for both parties to commit to certain behaviors that together constitute the core values of medical care. In the context of these fundamental ideas, it is easy to conceptualize the physician as an individual who would provide care for the sick by displaying compassion, commitment, and the expertise necessaries to tackle any human ailment, turn the clinical situation around, and ultimately restore the health of the patient if at all possible. In turn, the patient would be someone who was generally in need of healing, and whose behavior would make him

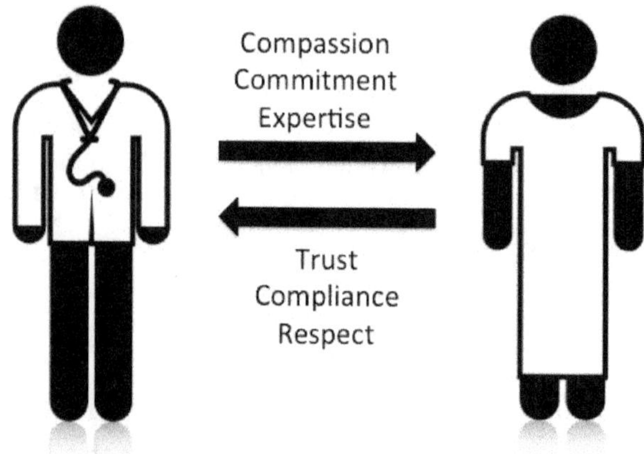

Figure 1-1
The Fundamental Physician-Patient Relationship

attentive, trustful, respectful, and compliant with regards to the instructions given by his physician. It is fair to say that, if either of them were to breach their covenant by deviating from these expected behaviors, the restoration of the patient's health would be compromised. The patient-physician relationship can be very simply illustrated by considering the two-way exchange of "vows" described above (Figure 1-1). Fair warning; I will continue to refer to this illustration throughout the book, as I modify it by introducing the various regulatory and cultural changes that have ended up distorting it, and by repeatedly pointing out how it is *this model* that should guide our analysis of the current state of affairs and our strategy for a possible solution to our problems.

To put it another way, I contend that, as a result of the intrusion of government regulations and consequent cultural changes, this simple relationship has undergone a progressive metamorphosis. I also submit that such influences have not made our healthcare better than it used to be (or less expensive) but rather more sluggish, costly, unfocused, poorly prioritized, somewhat corrupt and, yes, even fascistic. What once was a simple one-to-one relationship between physicians and patients is now an incredibly convoluted set of intertwined relationships that hardly resembles the original blueprint. Generally speaking, the changes that have affected healthcare revolve around the insertion of different organizations, policies and individuals between patients and their physicians. As the gap between the two original parties increased in response to such hurdles, the nature of *American Medical Exceptionalism* became replaced with an ever-expanding bureaucratic and impersonal system, one that lends itself ideal for downgrading. The common denominator of all these changes is the constant interference with the clinical decision-making process, typically by individuals without the qualifications to properly gauge the depth or appropriateness of such decisions and without an inkling of interest in taking the ultimate responsibility for the well being of the patient.

Enter third-party payers (Figure 1-2). We begin our account of the downgrading changes that have taken place along the contemporary history of American medicine with the introduction of third parties whose purpose has been to provide payment for the medical services rendered. Prior to this, and in line with the fundamental principles described earlier, physicians would provide services without considering compensation as their primary goal in life. In those days, patients' payment for medical services was often commensurate with their own financial capabilities, and the cost of care was relatively low. I still remember working in places where physicians were commonly paid in kind, or

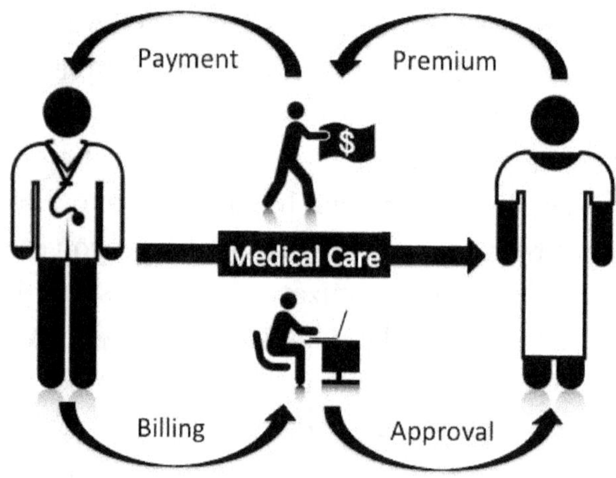

Figure 1-2
The Effect of Third-Party Payers

tangibly with goods that made the interaction with their patients look more like bartering. In the United States, the financial counterpart of such freedom of exchange was a fee-for-service system in which the compensation of the physician was proportional to the services being rendered. Within this framework, physicians were free to change their fees at will, using their own discretion and judgment to assess the impact of those fees. Such freedom assured, in part, the existence of a free market that responded to the laws of supply and demand. As a consequence, physicians were not viewed as a commodity, and those with the best results and reputation could charge more for their services, while those who provided lower quality service would be slowly ostracized by the patient population; a topic we will discuss further in the chapter addressing physician compensation. In those days, the inability of a patient to pay for a service was not necessarily followed by financial castigation, or purposeful withholding of the medical services needed. It was also very feasible for physicians to provide services at no cost to the patient when issues of professional courtesy were involved, or when it was very clear that the patient simply could not afford the services. In essence, without any strict set of regulations, those that could afford care informally subsidized the care of those that could not. This traditional system mirrored the overall state of a society with little government intervention, in which charity and compassion were a matter of private citizens looking after each other.

The introduction of a third party whose primary purpose was to assure total or partial payment for medical services has led to a variety of openly evident problems. The first of these is that it afforded the third party payers the rights to participate, and often command, the decision making process relative to care that required payment. In other words, since they were paying for it, they had a say as to whether the care to be delivered was appropriate, necessary, and covered by the existing policies, irrespective of their lack of clinical qualifications to issue such opinions. This is partially illustrated in the bottom half of Figure 1-2. Although the illustration oversimplifies this problem, as we will see in the chapter on physician compensation, third party payers have achieve this role by making billing for physician services one of the most cumbersome, inefficient and painstaking tasks known to mankind; one designed to deny payment of services as often as possible, and based upon any and every excuse conceivable.

Not surprisingly, the worst offender in this area is the federal government, by virtue of how the Centers for Medicare & Medicaid Services (CMS) set the national tone of third payer interactions with providers and beneficiaries. From the perspective of the practicing physician, this problem is palpable on a daily basis, every time an insurance carrier denies payment for services. As we will also discuss later, the attitude of both physicians and patients to this state of affairs is perplexing and, in my view, has contributed to the perpetuation of the problem. Although the introduction of Medicare and Medicaid in the 1960s appealed to the masses because of the perception that a welfare approach to the delivery of medical care was "fair", history has proved that both of these organizations have failed miserably in promoting high quality medical management for the patients they cover. Furthermore, at the present time, they represent the most bureaucratic, ineffective, inefficient and costly of all of the systems that relate to the healthcare industry. When we consider the nefarious influence of CMS on all other health insurers, it is not surprising that all third-party payers repeatedly interfere with the relationship between physicians and their patients by setting regulations, rules, guidelines, and all sort of hurdles that result in delays of care due to bureaucratic oversight.

The second problem derived from the adoption of a third party payer system (partially illustrated at the top half of Figure 1-2) is that the patient was no longer responsible for the financial burden of paying for the services. Over the course of time, this meant that patients have become fairly ignorant of the costs of the transactions being made, or the appropriateness of decisions relative to those transactions. From this point of view, such change began to influence the growth of a society of medical entitlement, which pervades the current interactions between physicians and their patients. Again, it is important for the reader to understand that Figure 1-2, as it is shown, oversimplifies this problem (e.g. the figure does not take into account health insurance provided by employers and how they relate to co-pays). A

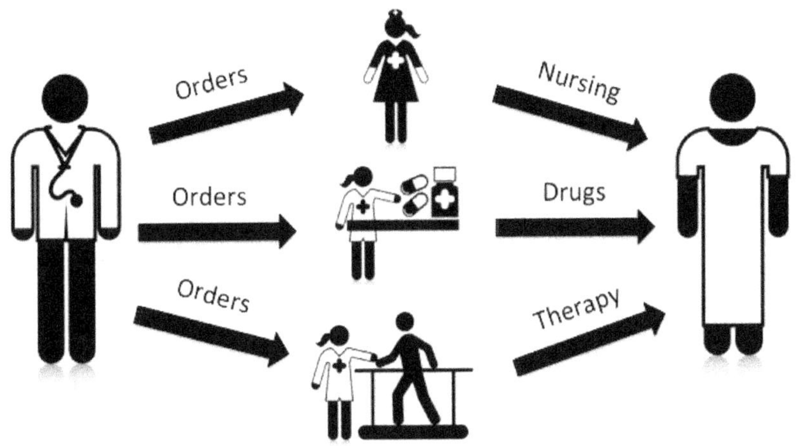

Figure 1-3
The Effect of Allied Health Professions

more detailed account of these issues will also be covered in the chapter on physician compensation. In addition, in the chapter on entitlements we will address the attitude changes characteristic of our society, and their manifestations and impact on the daily practice of medicine.

Enter the allied health professions (Figure 1-3). At the beginning of my career, I used to think of myself as a member of the physician community. At present, however, I'm commonly referred to as a member of the class of "healthcare professionals" or "healthcare providers". This departure from the traditional blueprint for my profession followed the introduction of a number of individuals with various degrees, who provide "ancillary" services that were never intended for the physician to deliver himself. It is practically impossible to consider medical care without somehow stumbling unto the ubiquitous cadre of nurses, therapists, nutritionists, pharmacists, technicians, or counselors, every one of them with opinions and views that may or may not be aligned with those that we consider appropriate for each clinical situation. Undoubtedly, Figure 1–3 also represents an oversimplification of the issue being discussed and it is clear that these individuals fulfill necessary roles in the care of patients, particularly those affected by complicated medical conditions. Furthermore, I am not oblivious to the need to involve these intermediaries in the various aspects of complex medical care as a result of the technologic evolution of the last three decades. However, the problem is that the cultural changes that have accompanied the introduction of all of these allied health professions have translated into their increased voluntary and extemporaneous participation in the clinical decision-making process, regardless of whether their qualifications warrant such a role or not. As we will see in the following chapters (particularly the ones on physician and nursing leadership), the problem with this paradigm shift is, at a minimum, the confusion created by communicating inaccurate or oversimplified concepts and opinions to the patients. Furthermore, increasing involvement in the decision-making process without a concurrent increase in the ultimate responsibility for the well being of the patient seems quite unfair from the perspective of those of us who have to face the consequences of clinical outcomes.

Enter the families (Figure 1-4). Another major change observed over the last three decades, and in my opinion also a product of the ever-increasing entitlement philosophy of our society, is a shift in the behavior of the families of our patients. Although clearly a similar change has been observed in the behavior of the patients, we have to set this aside because of the fact that the patients are an intrinsic part of the original fundamental clinical relationship (Figure 1-1) and cannot themselves constitute an interference.

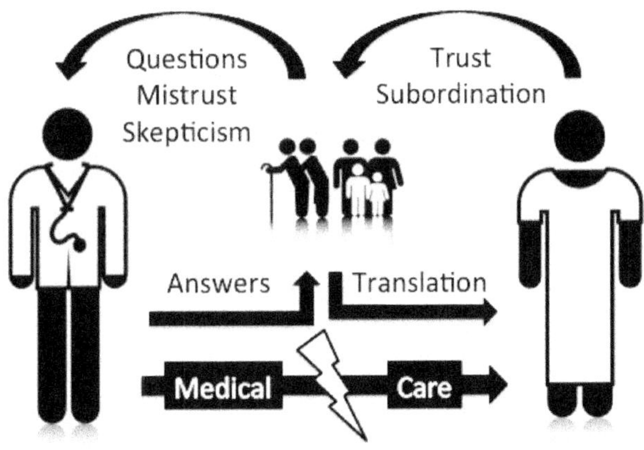

Figure 1-4
The Effect of Families

Nevertheless, it will be evident in the following chapters, that their behavioral changes must also be discussed in the context of entitlements. For the time being, however, we will only concern ourselves with the families and their role in directly impacting the fundamental principles. In the past, families constituted groups of individuals who seemed to be grateful for the care being delivered to their loved ones, eager to comply with instructions that were given to the patient, and willing to trust the judgment of the physician responsible for the management of their family member. Presently, on the other hand, it is not uncommon to experience how families come across as a mob of distrustful, self-centered, know-it-all, Internet searching individuals. As a result of this transformation, the point of care has gone from being the equivalent of a secular chapel, where the physician would hear the most intimate details of the patient's life and would do his best to restore health, to a battleground where every physician statement is questioned, doubted, challenged, and compared often with statements made by neighbors, acquaintances, or simply, heard in television shows. Not a day goes by that I do not come across a family member who insists in answering questions I directly ask the patient, repeatedly interfering with the basic interview process, and forcing me sooner or later to ask them to wait until I speak to them. Not a day goes by that I do not come across a family member who insists that he MUST understand the exact mechanism of how an antiepileptic agent is going to prevent seizures, even though he has not a clue as to what cellular membrane ion channels are. Not a day goes by that I do not come across a family member who tells me how *"WE are not having as many headaches"*, including himself with the patient as if the two of them represented a set of Siamese twins equally affected by the clinical process. Not a day goes by that I do not come across a family member that insists in translating every word I use to explain to the patient his clinical condition and treatment required, using terminology he picked up from unlikely sources and reflective of his own inaccurate understanding of the concepts being discussed; in doing so, he only contributes to the confusion instead of paying attention and trying to learn something useful. Sure, the reader will argue that these family members mean well and have the patient's best interest as their motivation for this intrusive behavior. Paraphrasing St. Bernard de Clairvaux, however, I submit that *"the road to hell is paved with good intentions"*, an aphorism that the reader is bound to remember repeatedly throughout the book in similar contexts. Moreover, my counterargument is that this is egotistical and self-centered behavior, wholly disrespectful of the patient who in most cases is not mentally incompetent by virtue of age or mental illness, and who should always be considered the most

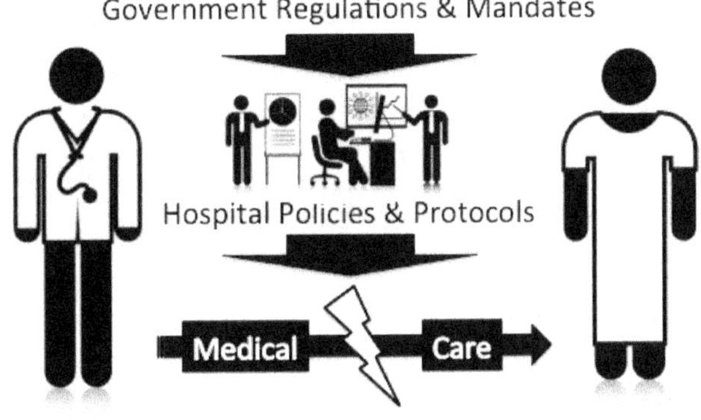

Figure 1-5
The Effect of the Bureaucrats

important individual in the clinical encounter. From the practical perspective, the energy required to discuss issues related to the healthcare of our patients with their families has increased at least five fold and continues to get progressively more exhausting. We will cover more in depth this whole topic in the chapters that follow, particularly the one on entitlements.

Enter the bureaucrats (i.e. politicians, government regulators, hospital administrators) (Figure 1-5). We could not even begin to discuss the downgrading of our healthcare system without giving a starring role to all the bureaucrats that run it. The individuals who make decisions about how the system is mandated to operate, the metrics that will be used to monitor its performance, and the accountability that lower level bureaucrats are to be subjected to in case of non-compliance with the mandates. Make no mistake, despite their grandiloquence, their interest is not the benefit of patients; it is all about power and control! Their control of the system; their having a say on how things are done; their telling the rest of us how it is going to be! Their arrogance is only matched by their greed, not only financial but societal, as they nurture their self-importance within the community they claim to serve. As we will see, their mere existence comes with a very high price tag; one that is painfully tangible when we consider the overall inefficiency and outrageous operating cost of that white elephant we call our healthcare system.

The interference caused by the bureaucrats on the fundamental process of the patient-physician relationship (Figure 1-5) is perfectly exemplified by the overreaching achieved by hospital administrations. Many years ago, when physicians were legally allowed to own hospitals or clinics, there was an automatic alignment of the priorities relative to the delivery of care. As the system has continued to evolve, however, hospitals have become organizations led by bureaucrats, even if some of them actually hold medical degrees. The result of these changes is that patients are treated within an environment where priorities are often at odds with those of the physicians. Now, it is true that hospital administrators are subject to pressures that derive from other bureaucrats in the form of government regulations, or from organizations appointed by the government to oversee their operations (see Chapters 11 and 14). However, in the following chapters we will see how there is a widespread lack of imagination as to how to align the well being of the patient with the fulfillment of government mandates that simply increase the level of bureaucracy.

In summary, medical care has traditionally been based on a simple two-way relationship between the patient and his physician. As originally intended, this relationship is comparable to a marriage in the fact that each of the two parties possesses his own inherent attributes and responsibilities. However, the downgrading of our healthcare system has revolved around the introduction of individuals and regulations that have come between the physician and the patient in one way or another, widening the gap between them. The result has been the transformation of the fundamental relationship into a sluggish and inefficient system.

2

Evidence Based Medicine

"A system of beliefs that stresses the need for prospectively collected objective evidence of everything...

... Except its own utility!"

Thomas P. Bleck, MD
Professor of Neurology, Neurosurgery & Critical Care Medicine
Rush University Medical Center

The publication of my colleague Tom Bleck's editorial on evidence-based medicine (EBM), from which the excerpt at the beginning of this chapter is taken, embodied a general sentiment among senior physicians (myself included) regarding the inadequacy of this discipline to provide a satisfactory pathway for the practice of high-quality medicine. Such position, clearly unpopular, and by some considered nothing less than heresy, must be critically examined. At the same time, we must look at the historical record of EBM since its introduction as a "revolutionary" philosophy to improve the delivery of medical care. I address this topic early in the book because there is no other aspect of medicine that, in my opinion, has been the subject of greater distortion since its introduction, and has been capable of changing medical thinking to a degree that we consider downright dangerous.

The concept of EBM, as well as its connotation as a departure from traditional ways of diagnosing and treating illness was introduced in our Country in the early 1990s. The basic premise was that, up to that point, medicine had been practiced based upon the opinion (expert opinion if you will, but more of this to follow) of physicians, and that such an approach was wholly inadequate because it included the inherited biases that each physician had developed over the course of his personal practice, based upon his experiences (i.e. hindsight bias) and points of view (i.e. confirmation bias). The early champions of EBM were quick to point out that the "emotional" dimension of such an approach to diagnosis and treatment left a lot to be desired and that a more objective, and hopefully quantifiable, method for assessing the existing information that could impact medical care was necessary.

Thus, a new way of thinking, characterized by giving prospectively collected data a premium place in the algorithms for clinical reasoning and decision-making processes was proposed. Unfortunately, the introduction of EBM was not accompanied by a thoughtful assessment of the potential unintended consequences that it could bring. In particular, there was a gross underestimation of the prevalent intellectual laziness within the world of clinical medicine (see Chapters 4 and 13), which promptly translated the basic principles of EBM into an oversimplified, monochromatic, and rigid dictum: *Without prospective, randomized, double-blind, clinical trials, it was simply impossible to reach sound clinical decisions about the treatment of patients!* In other words, prospectively collected data went from a premium place to an exclusive one. As we will see, this type of philosophy became the platform for the construction of "clinical guidelines", many of which currently threaten individualized clinical thinking and promote an environment of centralized control of medical care.

It is only fair that we begin our discussion by describing what was originally intended by EBM upon its introduction; and then contrasting the difference between the original plan and the distorted and erroneous discipline

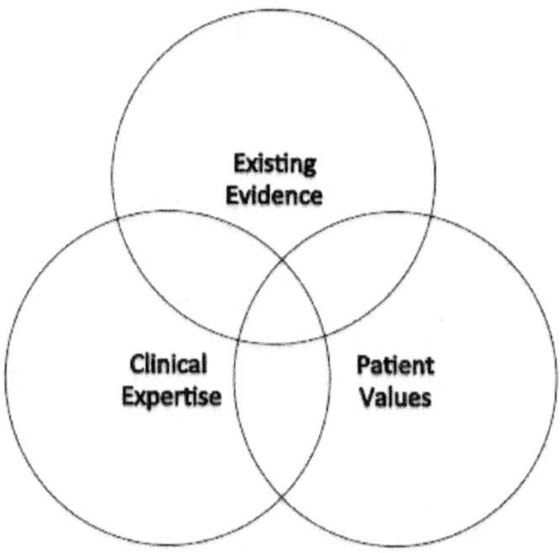

Figure 2-1
Relationship between the three original aspects of EBM

that it has become. The earliest champions of EBM comprised a group of thinkers at McMasters University, whose original purpose was to provide a much more comprehensive and balanced approached to medical decision-making. As such, they clearly stipulated that EBM was composed of three fundamental dimensions, which interacted with one another along the pattern of a Venn diagram (figure 2-1). This three aspects, or "pillars" of EBM, were listed as follows: The existing evidence (i.e. all evidence), the expertise required to assess the evidence (i.e. expert opinion), and the inherent personal values of each patient.

The first of these three was meant to encompass and take into account all existing evidence regarding clinical issues. It was never implied that only prospective or double blind data were sufficient or exclusive for making clinical decisions, as it is being interpreted at the present time in most clinical circles (particularly in the specialty of neurology). The authors understood that the word "evidence" is derived from the Latin term *evidentem* (i.e. "perceptibly clear"), in turn derived from *videre,* meaning, "to see". As such, it becomes readily apparent to any reasonable observer that there are different forms of evidence, each one with a different degree of strength but also bound by the reality of the type of information that can possibly be acquired under specific circumstances. From this point of view, there is no question that prospectively collected information is likely to be more objective than that which is acquired by retrospective assessment, the latter being subject to contamination due to the inherent inaccuracy of remembering information from the past. Does this mean that retrospective information should be discarded? Forgotten? Ignored? I think not!

I argue that all information is important, and that the so-called "evidence" is nothing more than a point within the continuum of certainty (figure 2-2). In this context, I further argue that, while there are concepts in medicine that are completely certain, incontrovertible and widely accepted, at the other extreme lay others that escape our understanding completely, or are unproven. Finally, I submit that approximately 80% of the topics and decisions made in daily clinical practice belong somewhere between these two extremes. With this in mind, it should not be surprising that, despite prospective data appearing on the surface to be stronger, they are not perfect!

Let's examine this point a little further. Together with the introduction of the idea of EBM, the notion that statistical soundness was necessary in order to validate the information has become one of the most misused tools in clinical discussions. It has, in fact, evolved into an obsession that rigidly limits our clinical imagination and, at least in my opinion, hinders the practice of good medical care. Not long

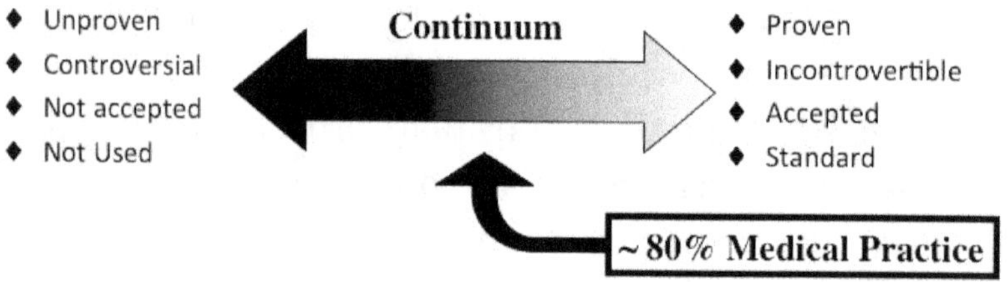

Figure 2-2
The Continuum of Certainty

ago, for example, in a cyber discussion between a group of stroke neurologists (i.e. the "experts" in our field) I was puzzled to see in my computer screen the following commentary relative to choosing the best course of action in the care of a patient whose case was being discussed:

> *"Since we don't have any data, we do not know what needs to be done"*

Granted, the individual making such a comment was a junior physician, but his statement left me wondering whether this person could find his way out of an elevator even if the doors were open. Discounting, of course, the possibility that someone were to present him with empirical data about the subject, or guidelines about the best process to exit elevators! Seriously? Have we abdicated our clinical reasoning? Have we become so intellectually lazy that we cannot practice medicine without a set of instructions? As we will see when we continue to discuss related topics (particularly medical education and leadership) later in the book, a statement such as that one is the tip of an iceberg constituted by the fundamental change in the role of physicians' intellect in clinical decision-making. An iceberg of a magnitude sufficient to sink the Titanic ten times over.

The problem is compounded by the mischaracterization of statistics as a source of quantification and objectivity. Alas, the tool to rescue us from the more traditional qualitative and subjective practice of medicine falls short of such expectations. In fact, those of us who have studied mathematics in a measurable way are somewhat taken aback by such inference, particularly when one considers the fact that mathematics is all about exactitude while statistics is all about probability and approximation. Therefore, it seems unreasonable to assign the virtue of absolute clinical certainty to the results of any study, regardless of how statistically valid they are. A clear example of this position is epitomized by the six months of critical editorial letters and rebuttals that follow the publication of any major prospective randomized double-blind study. We live in an environment in which we witness the daily publication of papers that take advantage of statistical analyses that support politically correct opinions and further academic careers, irrespective of logic and reason. In this milieu, we myopically look at these results, ignore all previous observations, and we congratulate ourselves in the use of this information under the premise of EBM.

Let's illustrate the subject of logic and reason before continuing our discussion. I ask the reader to imagine the statement: *"In the tropics, it rains frogs!"* Ludicrous as this hypothesis may sound, it should be possible to design a study that "proves" it (Figure 2-3). All you would have to do is

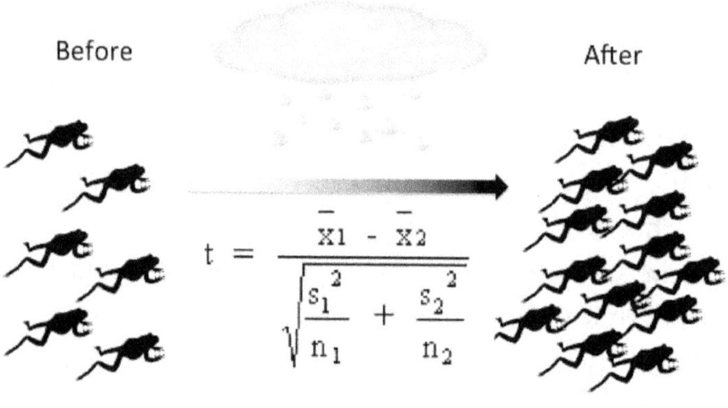

Figure 2-3
The Statistical Proof of Frog Raining (T-test)

count the number of frogs on the sidewalks before and after a storm (or a predetermined number of storms if you want to increase the sample size and the statistical robustness of your study), then subject the before and after results to statistical analysis (T-test statistic for example) to prove the validity of your original statement. Although no one in his right mind would waste time conducting such a study, I would predict that the difference between the counted frogs would be... ...wait for it... ..."Statistically significant!" Really?

The lesson to take away from our example is best illustrated by a quote popularized by Mark Twain: *"There are three kind of lies: lies, damn lies and statistics!"* However, this lesson seems to have fallen on deaf ears, as evidenced (ironically) by the growing number of medical statements based on statistical analyses that defy logic and reason. Additional examples of the disconnection between the obsessive need for prospective data and the application of logic and reason can be found in the literature. For instance, Smith and Pell's review of the empirical proof that wearing a parachute while jumping off an airplane leads to a decreased risk of traumatic injuries and death. Imagine that!

Another aspect of the idolatry presently practiced with respect of the use of statistics in medicine is the lack of understanding of the differences of the weighted impact of positive and negative results. Let me explain. Any medical study, particularly a therapeutic trial, that leads to a "strong statistically significant" positive result (e.g. the treatment is clearly better than placebo) automatically, and despite the impossibility to generalize its results as we will discuss later, has an overwhelming positive impact on medical care. Conversely, a negative result cannot be automatically assigned the opposite negative impact. The reason is very simple: There are many possible causes for such a study failing to show a benefit even though there is one! The most common of these are wrongful expectations, wrongful assumptions, wrongful execution, wrongful analysis, or any combination of these. In other words, the study was negative *under the conditions in which it was conducted*, not just under any circumstance. Therefore it is fair to say, just as William Cowper noted, *"Absence of proof is not proof of absence!"*

Now, we cannot let the "positive studies" off the hook either. As I noted earlier, their impact is much stronger particularly if the research methodology has been sound. A perfect example of this was the study that the National Institute of Neurologic Diseases and Stroke (NINDS) originally conducted to assess the effectiveness of using TPA (a so-called "clot-busting" drug) to treat acute stroke patients. Despite some of the criticisms along the way, the results of the NINDS study were very positive and its strength was such that it became a milestone in the realm of neurologic therapeutics. Still, the mistake that is commonly made when it comes to "positive studies" is the indiscriminate generalization of their results followed by their rapid inclusion in treatment guidelines. This problem stems from a failure to recognize two fundamental statistical concepts: 1) the relationship between the characteristics of the sample population and those of the general population, and 2) the constraints introduced by the details of the design of the study. The first of these essentially means that, in order for the results of any study to be applicable in clinical practice, the sample population (i.e. those patients treated in the study) must have identical clinical characteristics to the patient population for which treatment is intended. The less this relationship is true, in other words the less similar the sample population and the target population are, the less likely the results of the study will be applicable in practice. Therefore, to blindly apply the results of any study to a patient whose clinical characteristics are materially different from those included in the study makes absolutely no sense, and is likely to lead to unexpected results. The second of the concepts listed above refers to the circumstances in which the study was conducted. For example, timetables, doses of medications, allowances for concurrent treatments, and so on. Any deviation from the conditions in which the original study was conducted will introduce an element of contamination that may influence the outcomes. Interestingly, as strong as the results of the TPA for stroke patients study quoted above were, its application in clinical practice is a perfect example of the fundamental breach of both of the concepts described. Let me expand on this example.

The NINDS TPA study was conducted in a group of selected medical centers across the country, by specialists whose expertise and tenacity clearly qualified them as the best of the best in our field. Moreover, the patients included in the study were selected from the general population based on very strict criteria. Therefore, the study had positive results despite the fact that it was conducted under very tight conditions. A consequence of these conditions was that only a very small percentage of all patients who were considered for participation in the study were actually included. This, in and of itself is not unusual for a study of this caliber and magnitude. However, what followed the completion and publication of the study results was one of the most illogical frenzies witnessed to date in medicine. The neurologic community in general gleefully chanted statements such as *"Now we finally have treatment for stroke!"* and *"The treatment of stroke is TPA"*, essentially ignoring all other aspects of the care of these patients, and the many other practical therapeutic measures we had been using for decades. In turn, the pharmaceutical company that manufactured the drug spent millions of dollar into supporting initiatives to use TPA, mesmerized by the prospect of administering the drug to the 750,000 new strokes that occur every year in our country. Then came the disappointment. No matter how much effort or money was invested, only a small number of stroke victims were receiving TPA. How could this be? Clearly it had to be lack of education! So, more money was poured in! Physicians were educated, nurses were educated, and the public was educated. The proportion of patients receiving TPA only increased marginally. Puzzled? Most of the players in this drama were. Now let's look at this critically (Figure 2-4): First, we prove the benefit of a medication by testing in the best of the best medical centers, by the best of the best specialists, in a small minority of patients selected using very strict criteria. Then, we intend to treat patients from the

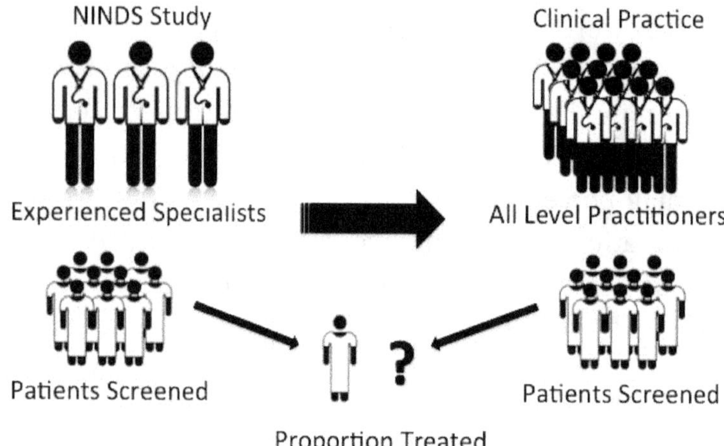

Figure 2-4
The Application of the NINDS Study in Practice

general population selected using THE SAME CRITERIA than those in the study, in the hands of every other physician in every other hospital without nearly the experience of the NINDS investigators, and we expect that we will be able to treat a larger number of patients. Are you kidding me? It makes no sense!

Adding insult to injury, not content with our obsession with the gullible use of statistics, we spread conclusions based on them as if they were gospel. In pursuing this course of action, we blatantly ignore the second tenet of EBM. It is clear to anyone with common sense that it takes a certain degree of expertise to be able to analyze all of the available information regarding a clinical topic, and to decide if and how it applies to a specific patient. Subjective and qualitative as this behavior may be, the originators of EBM recognized that it is practically impossible to apply the same information to every single clinical scenario and have similarly successful outcomes. I admit that I am quite fond of this aspect of EBM, probably because it validates the years of experience that I have in the practice of medicine. However, I ask the readers to ponder whether they would feel equally comfortable with having their clinical condition managed by a specialist with over a decade of experience, or by a young physician that just finished postgraduate residency. Again, it is not my intention to imply that junior physicians are less competent or less capable than those of us who have been around for a number years. But it is a fact of life that there is no substitute for experience, and this principle will have a significant bearing upon our discussion of other topics within this book, including physician's education, leadership, and the exchange of information with patients and their families.

Finally, even if we were to gather the best information available and analyze it based upon the best clinical experience available, the decision-making process would not be complete without considering what the patient himself wants and how he views his quality of life. This is, in fact, the third aspect of EBM and curiously the most prone to be affected by subjectivity. From this point of view, if the whole purpose of EBM was truly to change the practice of medicine to a completely objective and quantitative discipline, it would have to necessarily ignore the wishes of the patients. Just like anything else in our discussion, however, this can also be the subject of distortion since it allows physicians without sufficient expertise to hide behind options of treatment while forcing patients to make a decision that may be anything but informed. The truth is that everything we do in medicine carries a price tag, and there is no free lunch! It is impossible to offer chemotherapy to a cancer patient without also including the potential side effects attached to it (I will cover this further in Chapter 20), or to have a patient consider having coronary bypass surgery without factoring all the potential complications of such a procedure. In my experience, every patient has a different approach to making this type of decisions, in many cases seeking "second opinions" on his own, a subject I will cover in Chapter 18. Therefore, the outcomes of similar clinical scenarios are not necessarily going to be identical by virtue of several factors, not the least of which is the patient's views about his own life's outlook.

All these issues considered, and from the operational point of view, we should be able to combine all the three dimensions of EBM in order to have a balanced application of this discipline at the bedside; the way it was originally intended to be (Figure 2-5). But wait! If you look carefully at the illustration, you should quickly figure out that it is nothing more than a more detailed expansion of the fundamental patient – physician relationship that we introduced in the previous chapter and illustrated in Figure 1-1. Thus, should the medical community have paid attention and embraced the entire original concept of EBM (and not just succumb to the luring obsession with prospective studies and statistics), its foundation would have been so solid as to avoid the downgrading process. Instead, what is today commonly referred to as EBM brings only a diluted and unpalatable version of this discipline, as well as an oversimplified and lazy approach to medical practice: *Find a randomized prospective study for every decision you want to make in medicine, and do what it says!* Sadly, the popularity of this behavior is astounding, and the fact that it is being adopted at nearly every level of medical education is downright scary as it underscores the potential conformism and unsophistication of the physicians of future generations, those that will have the responsibility of caring for you and me as patients.

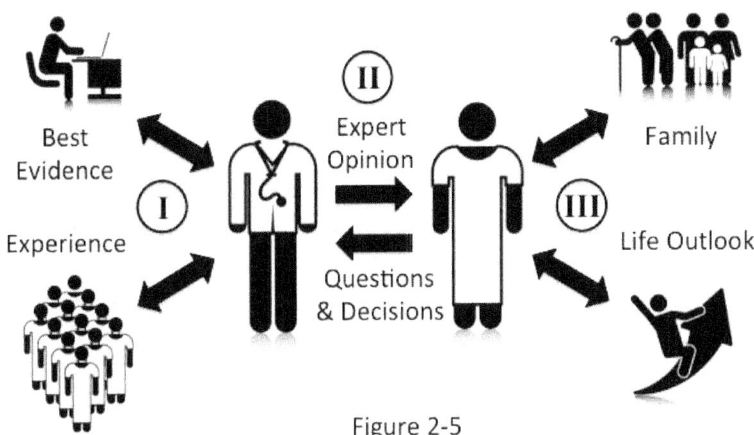

Figure 2-5
Original (Intended) Operational Blueprint for EBM

After all is said and done, however, the most dangerous aspect of the current popular version of EBM is that it has become the banner for the intellectual laziness that fosters the ever escalating compulsion for the insertion of Practice Guidelines in our daily lives. Their expansive dissemination virtually guarantees a progressively deeper government intrusion on the practice of medicine and, with it, further downgrading of its core values. Moreover, they strengthen the underpinnings of a culture of medical mediocrity that slowly creeps among us, infecting all aspects of the care of patients. Certainly, I am not the only one who feels this way or, for that matter, the most seasoned physician to have this opinion. My old friend Lou R. Caplan, one of the most experienced and respected voices in our specialty, has published extensively in this subject and has shown us the perils of having government agencies (or their surrogates) use treatment guidelines as a tool to make decisions about reimbursement or to grade the quality of medical care being delivered. In fact, these considerations alone do not begin to scratch the surface when we take into account the medico-legal implications of following or not following published guidelines.

In summary, EBM was originally introduced with the intent of improving medical decisions by removing inherent physicians' biases. The premise was the utilization of prospectively collected data that could be quantified and subjected to statistical analysis in order to guide decisions. Interestingly, the present widespread application of EBM is a very diluted and oversimplified version of its original blueprint, which included all existing evidence, the physician's expertise, and the patient's values. This current version is wholly inadequate and threatens to further contribute to the downgrading of the system. It also lends itself for governmental regulatory utilization.

3

Problem Oriented Medical Diagnosis

"The whole is greater than the sum of its parts"

Aristotle
Greek Philosopher and Polymath
(384 BC - 322 BC)

How would you like to be thought of as a "bag of problems"? In the 1960s, Lawrence Weed, M.D. pioneered the concept of the "Problem Oriented Medical Record (POMR)". His original intent, ironically, was to introduce an element of logic and disciplined thinking to the exercise of making clinical diagnoses to improve the accuracy of such a medical task. I have absolutely no quarrel with this lofty goal. In fact, as you may have guessed from some of the passages in the previous chapter, I am a firm believer in the necessity to use logic and common sense for the sound practice of medicine. To this end, I support every effort intended to make this possible. However, like many other interesting ideas in the contemporary history of medicine, the original work of Dr. Weed was not safe from the development of unintended consequences, or its perversion by the lack of critical thinking. In the next few pages I would like to discuss (just as I did for the concept of Evidence Based Medicine) the differences between what originally was intended when designing POMR and the discipline that it spawned "Problem Oriented Medical Diagnosis (POMD)", and their current status including their misuse at the bedside and abuse by regulatory agencies.

The original premise was that physicians' minds were incapable of concurrently handling numerous medical issues brought about by patients, and that by beginning to identify them and cataloging them into "Problem Lists", it made the task of diagnosing diseases more objective, scientific, thorough and comprehensive. At least theoretically, this approach would introduce a higher degree of efficiency and effectiveness, making the physician's ability to identify and track specific problems soar to its maximum expression. Furthermore, it would transform the art of record keeping in such a way that it would allow the introduction of computers in what became the first attempt at generating electronic medical records (EMR); again, a very imaginative and promising departure from the state of affairs at that time.

Unfortunately, the term "Problem" was defined as *"anything that threatens the health of the patient"*. The looseness of this definition left this whole concept open to misinterpretation, and essentially became the Achilles' heel of the entire theory. In the first place, as it is presently utilized, the term includes symptoms (i.e. what the patient *subjectively* feels), signs (i.e. what the physician *objectively* finds by examination), syndromes (i.e. the combination of several symptoms and signs together), ancillary data (i.e. test results) and even specific diagnoses (i.e. disorders or illnesses). Conceptually, the difference between all of these is vast and, before POMD became popular, no one in his right mind would have thought to pile them all together in one heterogeneous list. In fact, I submit that it is paradoxical that a process that began with a sound logical foundation would include in its core architecture a term that bears no conceptual logic. Even if the reader is not someone adept to any of the health related professions, he should be able to predict that an approach such as the one described about the utilization of the term *"problem"* is destined to lead, at the very least, to confusion and inaccurate medical documentation. However, as we will see, it has done far worse than that.

Let's explore this further, and start by pointing out the fact that it is perfectly conceivable that a patient's problem list includes the following:

- Headaches (Symptom)
- Fever (Sign)
- Meningismus (Syndrome of meningeal irritation)
- Leukocytosis (Laboratory showing increased white blood cells)
- Bacteremia (Diagnosis of bacteria in the bloodstream)

Now, anyone who has practiced medicine for any length of time should be able to look at that "problem list" and accurately make a diagnosis of *bacterial meningitis;* so, why the deconstruction? This question troubled me from the moment I set foot in our country to begin my postgraduate education. At that time, I had really not heard much about POMD because the educational style in my medical school followed the more traditional European model (Figure 3-1). As such, the way to make a clinical diagnosis involved a systematic identification of symptoms (via the clinical history, which accounts for approximately 90% the diagnosis) and signs (via the physical examination, accounting for another 5% of the diagnosis), and analyzing them in the context of the patient's risk factors and the temporal profile of the clinical condition (this analysis completed the remaining 5% of the diagnosis). At the end of this exercise, the physician was expected to generate a presumptive diagnosis, in essence a hypothesis that could be confirmed or rejected via ancillary testing (e.g. imaging, laboratory studies). This is in fact the method that I still use

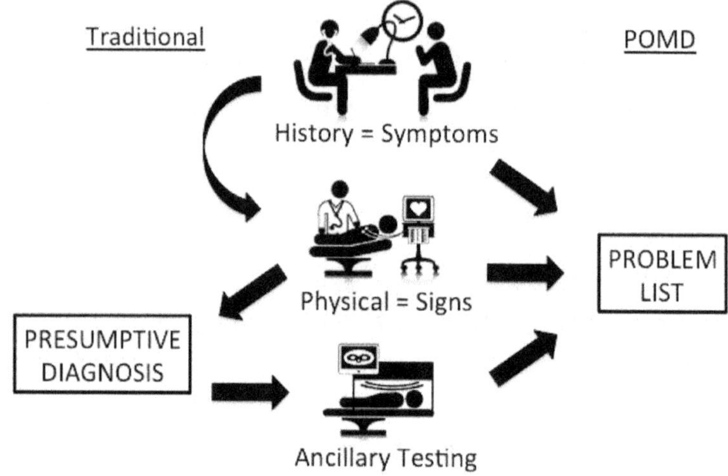

Figure 3-1
Difference Between POMD & Traditional Diagnosis

over three decades later, very successfully if I may say so myself. The downside of the traditional method I just described is that it requires for the physician to embrace the courage and willingness to be wrong. In other words, he must make a commitment; take a position; have an educated opinion based upon the equation:

$$CI + KE + DR = PD$$

Where CI = Clinical Information (Symptoms and Signs), KE = Knowledge and Experience, DR = Diagnostic Reasoning, and PD = Presumptive Diagnosis. At this point the reader may ask, *"How is this possible? Willing to be wrong? Doesn't that endanger the patient?"* Ah! You see, the system has an implicit clause that protects the patient while allowing the physician to assert his opinion. Let me explain.

The consequences of making an incorrect diagnosis are not all equivalent. They vary depending upon the diagnosis in question. For example, misdiagnosing a glioblastoma multiforme (an extremely malignant form of brain tumor with very short survivability irrespective of any treatment) does not have the same consequences as missing the diagnosis of pneumonia (a lung infection that is treatable with antibiotics and from which complete recovery is achievable). Based upon this difference, the traditional teaching has been that, *whenever more than one possible explanation for the patient's clinical condition is identified, they must be prioritized starting with the ones that are likely to cause the most harm if they are not properly treated.* This means that we are not concerned as much with the possibility of being wrong in our first diagnosis, so long as the patient is protected from the adverse consequences of an unattended and potentially damaging diagnosis. Let's share an example from my every day practice; that of patients who present with sudden dizziness, loss of balance, and often nausea with vomiting. Although the overwhelming majority of them will end up having nothing more than a temporary inner ear infection, the truth is that the most potentially devastating condition capable of causing this set of symptoms is also a precursor to stroke. Thus, we invariably treat these patients as if they are at high risk until we have fully evaluated them and have proved they are not in danger.

This is a safer approach, and one that takes into consideration the rules described above. Using this strategy, at least in this scenario, we could potentially be wrong 80–90% of the time. However, who cares so long as the remaining 10–20% of the patients are protected?

So, as I mentioned earlier, armed with this very different type of education, I came to this country and found myself wondering why we were deconstructing patients into problem lists rather than deductively looking for legitimate and prioritized diagnoses. After some time, I came to the realization that the reason for the widespread utilization of POMD, and the simultaneous departure from the method that by all accounts had withstood the test of time, was a combination of its ease and the promise of its contribution to an improved medical future. The latter promise, in my opinion largely unfulfilled, is a testament to how careful we should all be when invited to embrace any "new" strategy, rule, or method relative to the practice of medicine. I now would like the reader to take a closer look at Figure 3-1, in which I illustrate the fundamental difference between the traditional approach to clinical diagnosis and POMD. This difference is nothing but the deliberate an regimented *integration* of all available clinical information into the most reasonable diagnostic proposition, one that can be then tested by means of ancillary studies. This step, missing altogether from POMD (if not by design, certainly in practice) requires energy, discipline and experience, and therefore is not as easy to carry out as simply harvesting a group of "problems". Later in the book, when we discuss some of the problems we currently face in medical education (Chapter 4), I will point out the importance of integrative thinking for the clinician, and how it is slowly being replaced by a reorganization of the first two years of medical school curricula.

So, what difference does it make? Is this just another example of you say *"tomato"* and I say *"tomœto"*? I think not! As I mentioned at the beginning of the chapter, even a system that spawned from a reasonably good idea was not free from the danger of unintended consequences. These, in fact, represent the direct downgrading influences from POMD on the healthcare system. Although readily apparent, in my view these are not necessarily popularly discussed within the medical community at large. Nevertheless, they are tangible, ubiquitous, and of significant potential detriment to the patients under our care. Therefore, it is imperative that we address them, pull them from the shadows into the light, and recognize them for what they are: very negative aspects of the current healthcare system. There are three important unintended consequences, at least in my opinion, of the widespread dissemination of POMD: 1) The loss of deductive diagnostic reasoning, 2) The "multi-doctor gambit" and 3) Polypharmacy. I will elaborate on the first two in the next few pages, and I will briefly refer to the third since I have devoted a large portion of another chapter to it (Chapter 6).

Following along the lines of the incongruity I found upon starting my postgraduate education, I was perplexed by how intellectually uncommitted the medical students and residents were, and how everyone else seemed to accept this shortcoming as the *de facto* method for patient care. It would not be uncommon, for example, to read a medical record with a history and physical examination that began as follows:

History of Present Illness: This is a 25-year-old man who presents with a two-week history of headaches, nausea, visual abnormalities and no response to over-the-counter medications.

Then, after recording all of the remaining components of the history and physical examination, filling several pages, and following these with a listing of the pertinent laboratory studies that had been obtained up to that point, we would find the following entry in lieu of a diagnosis:

Assessment (Problem List):

1) *Headaches*
2) *Nausea*
3) *Visual abnormalities*

Seriously? As you can see, all the student did was to copy the list of complaints that the patient brought with him. There is a palpable intellectual failure to commit to a clinical diagnosis (in this case for example, "Migraine") with all the consequences this carries with it. The ability to process clinical information and derive meaningful diagnostic conclusions is not an innate skill. It must be learned and it must be polished through practice. Therefore, it is immediately apparent that, when students and residents are not held accountable to this intellectual process, it leads to a deficient subculture within the practice of medicine and it contributes to its downgrading. Presently, this problem has the weight of an epidemic; a rapidly spreading malady that infects everyone exposed and self-perpetuates as it negatively influences the integrity of the medical intellectual process. In combination with the changes being made in medical education (Chapter 4), it is guaranteed to progressively dilute the quality of physicians we graduate in the future, further contributing to a medical culture of mediocrity.

I could not find a specific reference to the nomenclature of the second of the unintended consequences of POMD, so I decided to give it a name myself: *"The Multi-doctor Gambit"!* The operational principle of this pervasive medical practice stratagem is based on a concept I first heard stated during one of my visits to the Mayo Clinic as an invited lecturer. Apparently, the philosophy on which that institution was founded included a view that *"If two heads think better than one, five think better than two."* This is tangible in the daily operations of the Clinic and highlights how patients are typically steered through the clinical services they receive. A patient is typically seen by a generalist who orchestrates the tests needed for diagnosis and makes referrals to all of the specialists that need to address the items contained in the patient's problem list. Sounds benign enough and probably reasonable. Doesn't it? The truth is that I have no objections to the conceptual need for specialists; after all, I am one of them! However, sometimes "more" is not "better", just "more". Combining the previously described consequence of POMD with this one could only have led to the outcome currently in evidence. Think about it, physicians do not have the intellectual need for making diagnoses but rather adhere to the complacency of constructing problem lists. So, what do they do with the problems in their list? They simply outsource them to other physicians, one at a time, for handling. Thus, the common scenario we currently see is that patients collect physicians to match each of the problems in their personal list. This scenario is particularly noticeable in hospitals, where many patients have one specialist per organ system, regardless of the reasons for admission. There are in fact physicians who insist on being the admitting physician of record for many patients seen in the emergency room, just to turn around and request multiple simultaneous consultations before they have even laid a hand on the patient. In our experience, we are commonly asked to see patients with "mental status changes" (Do not get me started on the worthlessness of this term) despite the fact that they are taking multiple mind-altering medications simultaneously. Shouldn't it be easier to just stop the drugs before calling more specialists into the case? Another scenario is that of multiple specialists being consulted for the same reason. This often leads to confusion and wasted time, particularly because of the uncertainty of who is responsible for what. Along these lines, I also think physicians commonly exhibit an existential problem: They don't seem to be content with *being* a physician unless they are *doing* something to the patient. This translates in every member of the "multi-doctor gambit" writing orders almost simultaneously and often without regard for the impact of their orders on the existing medical issues outside of their own scope. In the intensive care units, this represents a major problem; one that leads to back and forth conflicting orders or, worse yet, negative side effects. They order drugs that interact with one another and contribute to polypharmacy (see below and Chapter 6), request tests that lack prioritization and lead to scheduling conflicts, or simply make treatment changes that negatively impact other aspects of the patient's care. Sure, the supporters of the "multi-doctor gambit" philosophy contend that physicians should be able to communicate with one another and work in concert. However, I can assure you that this is easier said than done and, in practice, it seldom works.

The third unintended consequence of practicing POMD is polypharmacy. If we are to think of patients as problem lists, and we treat these problems independently, the result is that for every problem there will be a pill. It is important to recognize that one of the biggest problems we presently face in clinical medicine, particularly neurology (since many of the side effects we will discuss alter brain function), is the algebraic summation of side effects from the numerous concurrent medications the patients take. Therefore, from the point of view of our present discussion I must point out that, on following POMD, physicians are likely to prescribe medications that individually will take care of every "problem" the way this practice style intends for them to do. Unfortunately, having checked every item in the problem list as being "addressed" by pharmacologic means compounds the likelihood of the patient experiencing undesirable side effects. I will cover his in detail in Chapter 6.

Unfortunately, the downgrading effect of POMD does not end at the bedside but expands into regulatory hindrances. As we will discuss in Chapters 14 and 23, the latest governmental intrusion on medical practice derives from the American Recovery and Reinvestment Act of 2009 (ARRA), also known as the "stimulus bill". This legislation included funds to be spent in providing incentives (or bribes if you will) to providers and facilities that demonstrate their *"meaningful use"* (MU) of electronic medical records (EMR). Let me just point out that one of the so-called measures of MU, and a criterion for receiving financial incentives, is the electronic maintenance of on-going problem lists for patients. Sadly, even someone like myself, who is vehemently opposed to the utilization of such lists, is forced to do so by virtue of the fact that only government certified EMR vendors can be used under the MU program. Therefore, as you could have easily guessed, since the government makes the rules, and also certifies the vendors, it is practically impossible to find EMR software that does not include a compulsory problem list. Certainly, the one we currently use in our practice does! In our case, this has forced me to spend a considerable number of hours reprograming the software in such a way as to allow me to include clinical diagnoses only in my patients' problem lists. This is not necessarily an easy task, and certainly not one that most physicians are either interested or capable in accomplishing, particularly since the value they place on their time is probably quite different than mine. In chapter 7, as part of our discussion on physician compensation, we will cover the hurdle created by the International Classification of Diseases (ICD) codes due to the often-peculiar nomenclature that they use. Their inclusion within the system of POMD has in fact resulted in many terms being assigned a code when in fact they do not under any circumstance constitute a diagnosis (Table 3-1). The problem is compounded by the fact that the official acceptance of such terminology leads to additional consequences of its own, particularly when school dropouts or their equivalent are in charge of "pre-certifying" diagnostic tests and therapeutic procedures based upon "acceptable indications" that are found in lists plagued with non-diagnostic "problems" that experienced clinicians would never use.

Code	Description	Problem Category
338.1	Acute Pain	Symptom
344.1	Paraplegia	Sign
536.8	Dyspepsia	Syndrome
276.0	Hypernatremia	Laboratory Result

Table 3-1. ICD codes that are not real diagnoses

In summary, the introduction of POMD appeared at first to improve the ability of physicians to handle large amounts of diagnostic data by categorizing them so they could be analyzed more efficiently. Like many other great ideas, however, POMD fell prey to unintended consequences and is not in any way what it was originally designed to be. The three most important unintended consequences of the dissemination of this type of thinking have been the loss of deductive diagnostic reasoning, the "multi-doctor gambit" and polypharmacy, all of which significantly contribute to the downgrading of our healthcare system. Furthermore, the inclusion of POMD by government regulators as one of the criteria for the achievement of what they have termed to be "quality healthcare" has essentially intruded into the future of medical practices and has forced everyone who aspires to be part of the system to embrace such a dysfunctional concept.

4

Medical Education

"The first serious error we often meet... ...is the confusion of education with training... ...A genuine education enables one to acquire, for oneself, the skills one happens, at a given stage of one's life, to need. A training, on its own, contributes almost nothing to education and produces distressingly ephemeral advantages"

Peter J. Hilton
Distinguished Professor of Mathematics. University of Binghamton
In his foreword to "Mathematics from the Birth of Numbers"
(1923 - 2010)

The first time I read Professor Hilton's distinction between *education* and *training*, an excerpt of which I included above, it was almost as if the heavens opened and a beam of bright light shone on my head. Was that excessively melodramatic? Possibly, but I wanted to grab the reader's attention and force him to ponder about the important distinction made by his words. I must admit that I had never really considered the fundamental difference between these two terms and I suspect many others have not either. Yet, the contrast postulated in his writing explains, from a cultural point of view, some of the discrepancies I have witnessed in our educational system and didactic culture during my career. For example, something as simple as the term that we have traditionally used to refer to postgraduate residency programs (i.e. "training" programs) appeared in this context to leave a lot to be desired. Now, the reader may say, *"So, why all the fuss?" or, "What's in a name after all?"* Well, the conceptual disparity between "education" and "training" clearly embodies ongoing differences in didactic goals and strategies, both of which have led to outcomes that are quite unlike those that such programs originally intended. Along these lines, it is evident to me that we have approached this phase of medical education incorrectly. Moreover, additional scrutiny has led me to conclude that such a wrongful approach has counterpart distortions in earlier (i.e. medical school) and latter (i.e. continuing medical education) stages of the medical teaching experience. In the next few pages I will address the differences between what I consider to be the most important educational priorities in medicine, both substantively and stylistically, and those we currently accept as the norm. I will also discuss the implications, both present and future, for the changes being progressively introduced in American medical education by the *medical intelligentsia*, based upon disingenuous arguments that perpetuate the downgrading process that is carrying us to a mediocre medical future. I think the best way to start our discussion is by describing the process of medical education in our country, particularly because I suspect many of the readers may not be completely familiar with its various components (Figure 4-1). In addition, its extent, complexity and depth have a bearing on other aspects of our overall discussion, most notably physician compensation (Chapter 7) and leadership (Chapter 13).

In order to become a licensed physician, an individual must first be accepted to a medical school accredited by the American Association of Medical Colleges (AAMC) following at least two years, preferably four, of undergraduate college education. The pre-medical education requirements differ between medical schools but, at a minimum, must include one year of biology, one year of physics, one year of English

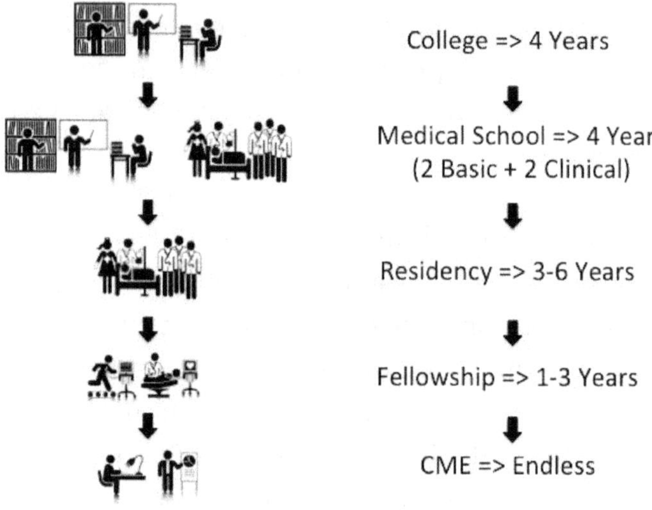
College => 4 Years
Medical School => 4 Years
(2 Basic + 2 Clinical)
Residency => 3-6 Years
Fellowship => 1-3 Years
CME => Endless

Figure 4-1
The Medical Education Process in the U.S.

and two years of chemistry (through organic chemistry). Acceptance to medical school is based largely on previous academic performance as measured by the individual's grade point average (GPA) and his score in the medical college admission test (MCAT). This is an incredibly competitive process, as evidenced by the small percentage of applicants that actually matriculate. A cursory review of 2011 data shows that the mean acceptance GPA score among US medical schools is never below 3.5 (Maximum = 4.0), while the mean MCAT score is never below 9 (Maximum = 15). After a minimum of four grueling years of graduate medical education, every student who is able to earn a medical doctorate then has to spend a number of additional years as a postgraduate "trainee" (i.e. internship and residency). The length of this portion of his education varies depending upon the specialty chosen. For example, internal medicine and pediatrics require three years of residency while neurosurgery requires six years. Finally, before going out as a practitioner, in certain fields of medicine there is additional subspecialty "fellowship training" required.[3] Fellowship can easily add 2 or 3 more years to the entire process (e.g. Interventional Cardiology). It is only then that the physician either becomes a faculty member in an academic medical center or enters the realm of private medical practice. Along the way, he must successfully pass the United States Medical Licensing Examination (USMLE), jointly sponsored by the National Board of Medical Examiners (NBME) and the Federation of State Medical Boards (FSME), and which is given in three separate parts that, in theory, respectively test a) basic sciences, b) clinical knowledge and skills, and c) the ability to integrate information for the practice of medicine. At present, all states rely on the USMLE to grant licenses to practice medicine. It is only after completion of all these steps that an individual can practice medicine unsupervised. But wait, we are not done yet, there still remains specialty (and subspecialty if necessary) certification by the chosen specialty board. This is independently conducted by each certifying board and can include both written and oral

---

[3] At present, accredited fellowship programs are also referred to as residencies but I have chosen to keep the older term for the sake of clarity

examinations. At present, board certification is generally time limited, with individuals being required to recertify every ten years or so. Finally, in order to maintain his medical license active, every practicing physician must accumulate a minimum of credit hours of approved continuing medical education (CME), which at present averages about 25 hours per year.

You would think after reading the previous paragraph that this process enhances the quality of the physicians that complete it; but does it? I submit that no process by design guarantees the quality of the outcome and I will expand on this point of view as it applies to topics in other chapters. Suffice it to say, my argument is utterly simple: *If process completion would unequivocally lead to quality, anyone capable of reading a cooking recipe would prepare dishes as good as those of Emeril Lagasse, Bobby Flay or Frank Stitt!* I additionally submit that the ability to complete and pass an exam is no guarantee of effective knowledge in the field being tested. Everyone knows that there are theories and courses designed to teach *how* to take exams successfully. More importantly, neither completing the educational process nor passing the exams guarantee *excellence!* After all, what do you call the person who graduates last in a medical school class? ...*Doctor!*

Finally, I would like to point out the financial burden that all of these educational and licensing steps place of any individual wishing to become a physician. Although I have chosen to cover this topic in the context of physician compensation (Chapter 7), let me just point out how much of a racket the medical testing system is. All the organizations behind these certifying tools (MCAT, USMLE, and Specialty Boards) charge astronomical sums of money for the privilege of vetting medical candidates at the different levels. In addition, individual state licensing boards also charge significant amounts for their licensing granting process. Working under the premise that they are stewards of the safety of the public, their "seal of approval" is sought and used to identify the chosen ones; and many wear it as a badge of excellence in medical practice. But, is it all of these things? Do we really believe that board certification makes a physician better? I have grown very skeptical that this is the case.

The devil is not only in the details but also in the emphasis that is placed on the priorities of the educational activities. Yes, if you peruse the website of the MCAT you are bound to read hyperbolic statements about how this test is designed to assess the candidate's *"problem solving, critical thinking and writing skills"* prior to acceptance into medical school. In turn, the USMLE claims to *"assess a physician's ability to apply knowledge, concepts, and principles, and to demonstrate fundamental patient-centered skills... ... that constitute the basis of safe and effective patient care"*. In my experience, passing these tests doesn't quite translate into possessing the qualities described. In fact, what I have witnessed over the last three decades is an increasing emphasis on students and physicians being able to quote published data and to cling to medical guidelines, rather than to critically apply sound clinical principles to individual patient scenarios. Contrary to such a "cook book" approach, and as I mentioned in the introduction to this book, I have instead favored the Socratic method of education during my years as member of two medical school faculties. I've always thought that, just like the proverbial *"give a man a fish and feed him for one day. But teach a man to fish and you will feed him for life!"* teaching students how to think is much more productive than asking them to regurgitate obtuse statistical analyses or the contents of "consensus statements". My argument is particularly true as the number of facts relative to any topic in medicine continues to grow almost exponentially, to a degree that makes it practically impossible to memorize (and remember) them all. Therefore, it appears more practical than ever to focus medical education on cultivating clinical discernment rather than preselecting the information some appointed committee considers "relevant" and applying it like automatons. However, this is not the current state of affairs, and hence the basic context for my forthcoming description of the major changes and trends I have witnessed in medical education over the last thirty years, from the graduate (i.e. medical school), through the postgraduate (i.e. residency), and all the way to the every day (i.e. CME) components. Along the way, I would like to impress upon the reader not only the downgrading effects of these changes, but also the increasing governmental intrusion and control behind them. Ready? Let's begin by considering the basis of medical school curricula, and the reforms revolving around them over the last two or three decades.

Themes
Integrating the Educational Continuum
Need for Evaluation and Research
New Methods of Financing
Importance of Leadership
Emphasis of Social Accountability
Use of New Technology in Education and Practice
Alignment with Changes in Healthcare Delivery System
Future Directions in Healthcare Workforce

Table 4-1. Themes for Medical Education Reform

After practicing medicine for many years, and analogous to Robert Fulghum's *All I Really Need to Know I Learned in Kindergarten*, I am convinced that all I really needed to know I learned in the first two years of medical school. You see, the traditional medical school curriculum, following Abraham Flexner's report of 1910, had U.S. students spent the first two years learning the basic sciences, mainly how the body is constructed (i.e. Anatomy), how it functions (i.e. Physiology), how it malfunctions (i.e. Pathophysiology), how is affected by illnesses (i.e. Pathology), as well as other subjects that together constitute the foundation of medical knowledge, including how drugs work (i.e. Pharmacology), how infective organisms cause disease (i.e. Microbiology), how illnesses affect families (i.e. Genetics), and how diseases affect populations (i.e. Epidemiology). The stronger this foundation is, the better anyone can use these central concepts to evaluate clinical situations and critically think about potential solutions. Trust me, not one day goes by in which I don't get to use some basic concept while caring for patients in intensive care units. For example, deciding the pertinent changes that need to be made in the controls of a mechanical ventilator requires implicit knowledge of pulmonary anatomy, physiology, pathophysiology, and pathology. However, I suspect my vision of the importance of basic sciences in clinical practice is not only unpopular but also hardly ever acknowledged. As I noted above, over the last 30 years or so, our country has witnessed a series of dramatic changes in medical school curricula. These have fundamentally altered how medicine is taught, all through the four years, but particularly in the first two. Although the proponents and supporters of such metamorphosis are chockfull of self-congratulatory statements, some of which have been published and can be found by means of a simple internet search, I remain unconvinced that we have made things better. Why? Well, for starters, common sense dictates that if it is not broken, there is no need to fix it! Therefore, in the face of the changes experienced, I suggest we explore them by attempting to answer the following questions: How come these particular changes? What has been their motivation? And, are we really producing better physicians?

The most important changes made to medical school curricula can be found in the existing literature organized around eight major themes developed by the National Advisory Panel of a conference jointly organized by the American Medical Association (AMA) and the American Association of Medical Colleges (AAMC) (Table 1). They include: 1) Integrating the educational continuum; 2) Need for evaluation and research; 3) New methods of financing; 4) Importance of leadership; 5) Emphasis on social accountability; 6) Use of new technology in education and medical practice; 7) Alignment with changes in the healthcare delivery system; and 8) Future directions in the healthcare workforce. In my opinion, this list of themes indicates that the entire process of medical education reform is designed rearward, with the changes suggested being subordinate to the existing or the predicted needs of the "healthcare system". Does this make sense? Not to me. The idea that we should modify our educational priorities and strategies just so they can fit the expectations of an already dysfunctional system simply makes no sense. This feeling of inappropriateness grows as one examines the specific changes being implemented. In all fairness, as I reviewed the available literature, some medical schools have made reforms that make more sense than others. However, some of the most egregious changes I found, followed by my counterarguments, include:

1) Exposing students to clinical experiences in the first two years. The students apparently have complained that they think it is not helpful not to be exposed to patients until their third year. Personally, I would not let students progress beyond their second year unless they mastered the basic sciences. As I mentioned earlier, I think the first two years are the most important of them all. I also think that sending a first or second year medical student to see patients, just so he can feel good about being a "student doctor" (see below) is similar to going to a foreign film that has no English subtitles! You may get a vague idea of what is happening, but you are liable to reach wrongful conclusions and, accordingly, act erroneously. I shriek to think that we are attempting to teach physical diagnosis to freshmen and sophomores who do not have a clue about what murmurs mean or what an internuclear ophthalmoplegia implies. I taught those courses and I remember the clueless looks and the lack of interest in their faces.

2) Integrating learning across disciplines based upon systems. On the surface, this appears to be a very smart idea. However, I submit that one of the most important qualities a physician must possess is the ability to integrate information from a variety of sources; in fact, probably *the* most important! Thus, if we prevent them from using such an attribute by changing the design of the curricula so the integration is programmatically achieved, soon we will be unable to discriminate those who are capable of truly practicing medicine from those

who simply do not belong. Another argument made on behalf of leaving integration to the individual is that developing curricula around it prevents redundancies. In my view, redundancies allow two things: a) Hammering important concepts in a way that facilitates their learning, and b) Provide the intellectual bridges for conceptual integration.

3) Tailoring the educational experience to the "societal needs". I find this to represent a slippery slope. It is often difficult to reconcile the needs of the individual patient with those of the society. I submit, as I have said throughout the book, that the fundamental patient – physician relationship (Figure 1-1) has to be the core of any meaningful system of medical care. Physicians are not sociologists or social workers and the so-called psychosocial concerns of patients should be prioritized based upon specific clinical situations and not based on populations. Furthermore, it takes time in practice and experience to learn to read the subtle psychological nuances of a clinical encounter, and such a skill cannot be readily taught in a classroom. Finally, it is precisely when we substitute the patient's needs for those of society that we open ourselves to the introduction of medicine *à la Carte,* a concept that has nothing but a downgrading effect on the daily practice of medicine.

4) Team building as a core competency. I have no argument with the fact that medical care ultimately requires teams of people to execute all aspects of it. My problem comes from the touchy feely notion currently disseminated that *"There is no 'I' in TEAM"*. I think exactly the opposite. As I will cover more in depth in Chapter 13, there can be no

functionality in any team without a captain! For better or for worse, only the physician is qualified to lead the team and, as such, he carries the ultimate responsibility (i.e. the burden of command). That places him in a very singular position, not to be shared by other "healthcare providers". Thus, unless we take this position in medical education, we are liable to produce generations of clinical pushovers who will not have the spine to stand up to regulators, bureaucrats, or simply counterproductive colleagues. I find it interesting that this has been one of the educational reform priorities since leadership development for physicians is also another, opening the interaction for potentially inadequate outcomes.

5) <u>Students must be taught about the healthcare system</u>. Even though I have no argument with teaching students about the system, the real issue is what message are we giving them. In other words, do we teach them how to adapt their behavior and performance so it fits the system? Essentially to acquiesce; or do we show them the correct path and allow them to compare it and contrast it with the current (or future) state of affairs? For example, one of the medical schools I reviewed now includes a program by which third year medical students go to Capitol Hill to "listen to politicians and experts debate the changing health-care system". Really? Do we want young, inexperienced, and impressionable minds to be exposed to the demagoguery and corruption spewed by the same people you and I painfully watch nightly in national television? I submit that they do not possess the knowledge and experience necessaries to gauge the accuracy of what is being said. Moreover, I suggest that programs like this are illustrative of the healthcare

system brainwashing currently being imposed on medical education, and which I will cover in greater detail later.

Now, the motivational forces for all of these medical curricula changes are explicit in the writings available on the subject, the most common being: Medical students feedback, complaints by the public about their physicians, and the appeals made by payers for healthcare insurance. All of these have been amalgamated into statements such as *"Society demands change in medical education!"* (Paraphrasing several of the sources reviewed). Seriously? The same society that insists in knowing more medicine than the physicians by surfing the Internet through sites such as WebMD (see Chapter 18) and that is full of entitlements (see Chapter 19)? Even if I did not know anything else, I would have predicted that revamping our medical education based upon the "needs" on any of these groups is a recipe for downgrading. Let's start with the medical students.[4] In principle, I find it irrational to have the students comment on the appropriateness of any curriculum *while they are still students*. How could they possibly know what they will need in the future? How could they possibly know what is relevant or not? They simply lack perspective, no matter what they think of themselves, or how smart they are. According to the champions of medical education reform, students *"object to being stuffed like turkeys during their first two years of medical school: They are taught about the most recent advances in the basic sciences which they cannot possibly absorb and much of which they will forget after they enter*

---

[4] Even though I have recently been informed to refer to them as *"Student Doctors"*, I find the latter term to be another unnecessary label change by the *"Human Fulfillment Movement"* and I am inclined to ignore it

clinical training". I find this line of thinking juvenile. I still remember when I was a child arguing the usefulness of being compulsorily taught about classic mechanics since it was unlikely that I would ever use any of these concepts in medicine. I can assure the reader that I could not have been more mistaken. For example, it is impossible to understand cerebral blood flow or vascular ultrasound without a working knowledge on fluid dynamics. So, the medical students argument is presumptuous and misguided, but I suspect effective because of the current climate of medicine socialization, the obsession with political correctness, and the overwhelming urge to please them and keep them happy (hence the new appellative of *Student Doctor*).

The role of the public in motivating medical education reform has been reported as that of a growing set of criticisms about physician's availability, communication skills, and their ability to provide effective counsel to the patients. I will discuss the bulk of these complaints in the context of other topics, specifically physician compensation (Chapter 7), malpractice (Chapter 9), leadership (Chapter 13) and patient entitlements (Chapter 18). Suffice it to say, however, there are two sides to this topic and I think, at least in some measure, the patients are justified in their criticism of physicians. My disagreement lies on the fact that such reproach does not necessarily point to the need for an educational reform but rather the opposite: The need to return and reaffirm the fundamental physician-patient relationship (Figure 1-1) as the core of the system of medical care. I am all for holding physicians accountable for their end of the clinical contract, which should take care of the bulk of the public's complaints. However, I think it is unfair and short sighted to even attempt to address these without factoring the financial, regulatory, and litigious pressures currently experienced by practicing physicians.

So, what about the medical education reform pressures exerted by the payers (including the government, private insurers, and employers)? Their contention is that the "escalating cost of healthcare" is closely related to inadequate education of medical students. In fact, every movement to remodel the healthcare system includes an educational reform section, destined to provide graduating physicians with what they call a set of "expanded competencies to allow them to function within the current managed care environment". Although I do not discount the need for physicians to be informed about the system in which they operate, the changes made to medical school curricula relative to this topic give the impression that the tail is wagging the dog. In other words, as I will show in other chapters, there is no doubt in my mind that part of the problems we currently have is the direct result of the physician community abdicating their leadership position in the medical care experience. Thus, is this what we are going to be teaching students? To acquiesce to the regulations without any thoughtful consideration? To "play the game" offered by a downgraded system without an ounce of spontaneity? To bow down to the *medical intelligentsia* without expressing an opposing opinion because of the risk of being labeled as a "disruptive physician"? In my opinion, medical school is not the time to introduce this type of education, except perhaps prior to graduation. Moreover, if it were to be done, the tone should not be one of servitude to the system, with the compulsion to blindly follow the processes irrespective of the consequences to the patient. I would like you to refer back to the difference in attitude I think is required of future physicians when perusing several of the other chapters, especially those focusing on paperwork, regulations, protocols and conflicts of interest.

Now that we have addressed the changes experienced by the medical students bound to be the physicians of tomorrow, let's take a look at what happens when they enter post-graduate residency programs. First let's discuss how it used to be, or the *"good old days"* if you will. Traditionally, residency was a war zone. Most major programs included rotations through clinical services in inner city, county or Veteran Administration (VA) hospitals, where the patient population was riddled with severe medical ailments; the sickest of the sick! As residents, we were expected to work long hours, take care of numerous patients, make sure the clinical services ran 24-7 so the attending physicians (i.e. our mentors) could spend their time teaching. The teaching ideally took place at the bedside or in the operating rooms depending upon the specialty chosen, sometimes both. We were accountable for every decision we made. Criticism was sharp, in our faces, but with scarce exceptions, not meant to be personal. Conversely, we were competitive, we wanted to excel, and we craved the praise of our elders for having performed up to their expectations. In fact, I distinctly remember the feeling of elation after uncovering an unusual clinical finding or making a difficult diagnosis prior to the attending physician having done so, gaining sometimes just a simple nod of approval. Yes, we were overachievers; there was a passion for excellence in our every day work, and not just the desire to complete the tasks assigned to us so we could mark a checklist. We understood that, by performing at our best, and by learning exponentially, we had a shot at the brass ring: Being appointed Chief Resident in our last year!

How long were our hours? Well, let me paint you a picture. When I rotated through the Medical/Coronary

Intensive Care Unit at the University Hospital in the early 1980's, each team was on call every other day. This meant that we would come in at around 7:30 am and make joint bedside rounds with the team coming off call from the previous day. We would then take over the unit patients, spend the night, and make rounds with the incoming team the next morning. These rounds would end approximately at 10:00 am or so, and then we would proceed to finish writing our clinical notes. Typically, this would take a couple of hours and, around 1:00 pm or so, we would finally go home. The next morning, we would be back again to start another identical cycle. This meant that every day we woke up in our own bed at home, we were on call that night! Excessive? One could argue that, but I am here to tell you that the learning experience could not be replaced by anything else. Coming out of that rotation we felt competent, efficient and confident, three attributes that greatly improved the odds for the very sick patients under our care. Now, in all fairness, not all my residency years elapsed according to this schedule. Most of the time, we were on call every third night. In those days, nearly all residency programs had a similar schedule, which meant that our workweek might span up to 120 hours. Excessive? At times we thought so too. However, in retrospect, the depth and width of our learning experience practically guaranteed that, at the end of our residency, we were capable of going into the community with minimal risk for the patients since we had accumulated mounds of supervised clinical experience in our field. By then, we had had ample opportunity to screw up within a controlled environment, having the safety net of several supervisors (i.e. upper residents, fellows and attending physicians), who hovered around us looking over our shoulder and modifying our every wrongful diagnostic and therapeutic decision along the way. Unfortunately, times have changed and not for the better. Let me explain by introducing you to Libby Zion.

In 1984, this 18 year-old woman was admitted to a New York City hospital, where she died a day later as a result of a clinical syndrome precipitated by drug interactions (i.e. the serotonin syndrome). The patient's father (a prominent attorney) took the position that his daughter had been "murdered" by overworked, negligent resident physicians and eventually convinced the district attorney to convene a Grand Jury to consider murder charges. Although the Grand Jury declined to issue an indictment, the residents eventually were found guilty in a number of counts of negligence, and were reprimanded. Although the State Court of Appeals eventually cleared the records of these physicians, the New York State Health Commissioner appointed a panel (known as the Bell Commission) that eventually recommended limitation of the residents' work hours. In 1989, the State of New York adopted this recommendation, and in 2003 The American Council for Graduate Medical Education (ACGME) adopted it as the new standard for ALL residency programs across the nation. This brings us to today. The two passages of the new set of regulations that I consider most relevant to our discussion are the following:

"Duty hours must be limited to 80 hours per week, averaged over a four-week period, inclusive of all in-house call activities."

And

"The program must ensure that qualified faculty provide appropriate supervision of residents in patient care activities."

Before we proceed to address the negative consequences of the first of these two statements, let me say that it is not my intention to defend the argument that it is acceptable for physicians to work when they are exhausted, or that medical errors should be condoned. On the contrary, just like any other aspect of human behavior, the *good old days* I described above had an inherent dark side, or a "blind spot" if you will. A schedule such as the one we used to hold, lent itself prone to abuse by all parties. And THAT was the problem, not the long hours *per se*. Let me expand by introducing yet another anecdote. During one of my last faculty meetings before I left the university, I was taken aback by what seemed to be an endless argument between several of my colleagues centered around the dilemma of whether the attending neurologist supervising the General Consultation Service in the hospital was required to round with the residents on both Saturdays and Sundays, or just one of the two weekend days. Mind you that, at that time, each of these faculty members rotated as supervisor of that service one month per year. So, here we were, arguing about working four extra days out of 365!

You see, in many instances the problem has really been the inadequate supervision by faculty members whose intellectual laziness had a physical counterpart. This behavior, common among the academic community, led to "dumping" the work on the residents and, at least in my opinion, placed every one of the parties at risk of suffering negative outcomes. I still remember how other faculty members in our department viewed my partners (the colleagues who rotated supervising our Vascular and Critical Care Neurology service) and I with certain contempt because of the different style in which we ran things. In our service the residents were required to discuss every major diagnostic and therapeutic decision they made with the attending physician on call, even decisions made in the middle of the night. This philosophy assured three things:

1) The patient benefitted because the decisions were not solely made by a junior resident, but sanctioned by the most senior and experienced member of the treatment team.

2) The resident benefitted because he received immediate feedback about the quality of his decision; this contributed to his education while it avoided the feeling of isolation and stress related to operating in a vacuum.

3) The attending physician benefitted because, after all, he was ultimately responsible for the patient's care. Therefore, he did not have to go through the process of having to undo decisions made in error without his consent.

It always appeared to me to be an all-around fair deal, and it worked! I submit that it was the failure to use this type of supervision strategy, not just the long working hours of the residents, that led to the catastrophic death of Libby Zion, as well as to the disastrous educational changes triggered by that event.

Yes, I know that there have been scholarly papers published in support of the argument that long working hours are associated with greater number of medical errors. However, without dwelling on the methodological shortcomings of these studies, I contend that errors are opportunities for learning (a concept widely embraced by the current *medical* and *nursing intelligentsia*) and, therefore, I would offer the following relevant questions relative to the dubious conclusions of their analysis:

1) Is residency not the best time to make errors that, under proper supervision can be adequately intercepted, and from which the resident can derive some learning? If not, when? Once the physician is practicing unsupervised?

2) Shouldn't supervising faculty members have the qualifications and experience to exercise discretionary powers that allow flexibility in resident's work hours that would prevent fatigue and burnt out? Isn't that, in fact, a part of their supervising duties? If not, do they really qualify as proper supervisors?

The answers to these questions provide the framework to critically examine the ACGME regulations, particularly those noted above. Let's begin by addressing the compulsory limitation of work hours. By now, the reader should be in a position to side with only one of two possible viewpoints about the reasonableness of this regulation. Either the *medical intelligentsia* is right, and we have been grossly overworked residents, or they are not. Guess what? I don't think it matters which argument is correct, since the result of cutting down residency working hours has been the same: Decreased learning! Think about it! There is a certain amount of material that must be learned and a number of patients to be treated under supervision, in order to gain the fundamental knowledge and experience necessary for becoming a specialist (i.e. an expert in a medical field). Traditionally, it has taken a very specific amount of time to acquire these skills. If we come around and decrease the amount of time available for learning by 30% (i.e. from an average of 120 hours per week to 80 hours per week), the product of the residency programs will be a physician who is about 30% less experienced. So, what we have done is displace some of this individual's learning process into his early practice, at a time when he will be unsupervised and will have no safety net. Is that what we want? Clearly, one could argue that the solution is to increase the duration of the residency programs to compensate. I can assure you that this is a very unpopular notion, and one that is bound to hurt specialties that already have lengthy postgraduate programs such as Neurosurgery and Interventional Cardiology.

The second of the ACGME regulations listed seemed baffling to me. If we now have to require that the supervising faculty be qualified to exercise such supervision, what were the previous requirements? And if the previous requirements were inadequate, doesn't that support my contention that the original problem was not the working hours but the inadequate supervision? Again, it seems that we are going around in circles. Yet, the current landscape of postgraduate medical education is one riddled with regulatory constraints and the consensus among my colleagues remaining within the realm of academic medicine is that the work hour limitations have been nothing but detrimental. Let me illustrate this point. A colleague of mine who is Professor of Neurosurgery in a Medical College of the Southeast describes how difficult is making morning rounds with residents who know nothing about the patients because they just came in to replace the residents who admitted the patients the night before and have already been forced to go home because their allowed hours were up. Finally, I would also like to point out that, as part of this regulation, residents are now required to clock in and clock out, just like any blue-collar worker. Personally, I view this as part of the brainwashing described above, the indoctrination of physicians that is likely to shape them into public servants, puppets of governmental regulations at all levels.

I purposely left our final question about medical education reform, the one dealing with the quality of the product of our current system, to address it in conjunction with the quality of post-graduate residency graduates. The reason is simple; the behavioral changes resulting from both of these experiences are very similar. I must say that I have been somewhat disappointed by most of my recent encounters with residents and medical students. Barring a few exceptions, I have found them unjustifiably conceited, eager to conform to the system, prematurely critical, and with a sense of duty that leaves a lot to be desired. The most common scenario has been during a recruitment interview when they commonly leave me with the impression that they want to work short hours, take call infrequently, and make a lot of money. Wow! I would love a job like that too! They are happy to quote papers and guidelines, comply with every request made of them regardless of its legitimacy, follow rather than lead, readily agree rather than debate, and they are practically incapable of an original thought. In my view, the physician we are creating for the future is an hourly public servant who conforms to the needs of the system. This saddens me...

The final leg of our medical education, the one that we have to indefinitely experience in order to remain in practice is known as CME. The problem with CME is its heterogeneity, with some offerings being of excellent quality, other simply dismal, and many others somewhere within the spectrum. In my opinion, continuing life-long learning is a primary responsibility of every physician; a necessity similar to breathing. My problem is, again, with the regulations that rule the accreditation of CME offerings and their content. The fact that they emphasize the teaching of guidelines, consensus statements or government mandates (e.g. Food and Drug Administration approved information) has become a subtle form of censorship and brainwashing. They perpetuate the educational direction described earlier for medical students and residents.

In summary, medical education is a long and structured process that spans many years. Its purpose should be to produce physicians in all the sense of the word; individuals that honor the fundamental physician-patient relationship and are capable to be responsible for human lives. However, the last several decades have seen strong moves to reform the medical educational experience at all levels, not necessarily for the better. Change and evolution by themselves are good, notably when they address valid needs and concerns. However, change for the sake of change, or worse, relative to the perceived "needs" of a downgraded medical system, is likely to profoundly alter the quality of our physicians. Our current educational system, if unchecked, is bound to continue to produce the American physician of the future: An hourly public servant! Is this what we really want? Can we change this future? Keep reading...

5

Nursing Education

"Education is not the filling of a pail, but the lighting of a fire"

William Butler Yeats
Irish Poet and Playwright
(1865 - 1939)

I would be perfectly content if I never again had to hear the declaration *"I am a nurse!"* as a warning shot that pretends to imply that the person making it (typically a patient's family member) is sufficiently educated to understand anything I have to say about a medical subject. Harsh words? Possibly; but I assure the reader that behind their self-important and overconfident assertion, there is usually little substance. More often than not, the individual who so eagerly volunteers having such a credential has some vague or inaccurate notion of the subject at hand, clearly a product of a weak education supplemented by uncritical Internet searches; to quote the poet Alexander Pope: *"A little learning is a dangerous thing; drink deep or taste not the Pierian spring."* Despite what it may seem up to this point, I am not trying to belittle nurses because of some deep-rooted hatred of them so you can dispense with any unnecessary psychoanalytic effort. On the contrary; I am trying to get the reader's attention about one of the most important topics relative to the downgrading of healthcare: *The downgrading of nursing as a profession!* Let me first clarify that nursing is, in my view, one of the most important pillars of medical care. This is particularly true in hospitals, and especially in intensive care units. The truth is that we make rounds daily for a few fumbling moments, write some orders, and walk away, leaving nurses to execute every aspect of our treatment plan. Furthermore, nurses are our eyes and ears during the interval until the next time we see the patient, gathering information essential to the decisions we will be asked to make. Therefore, their importance cannot be overemphasized, and their inability to step up to the clinical tasks required of them carries with it grave consequences for the well being of the patients. Alas, the basis of this problem, as I see it, is that nursing is its own worst enemy. As we will discuss in Chapter 12, there is a serious deficiency of true nursing leadership in our country, and I argue that it begins during the educational process. I submit that the dysfunctional educational system currently in place for nurses, and sanctioned by the *nursing intelligentsia*, if examined carefully, yields no surprises and it could not have led to anything but the incompetent ethos we are currently experiencing.

Let's start by asking: What does it take to become a nurse? In the previous chapter we covered in substantial detail the path that leads to the making of a physician. Analogously, in the next few pages, I will address the issue of the educational requirements to practice nursing, emphasizing the significant differences between this profession and mine, as well as within the various components of nursing itself. It is important that we point out all of these differences because the public does not seem to understand them and there is a general tendency to consider nurses at an equal level to physicians. In my opinion, such a broad stereotype is wholly unfair to all parties involved. Before you think that my comments are arrogant or conceited, please bear with me for the next few pages, in which I will also point out the reasons for my points

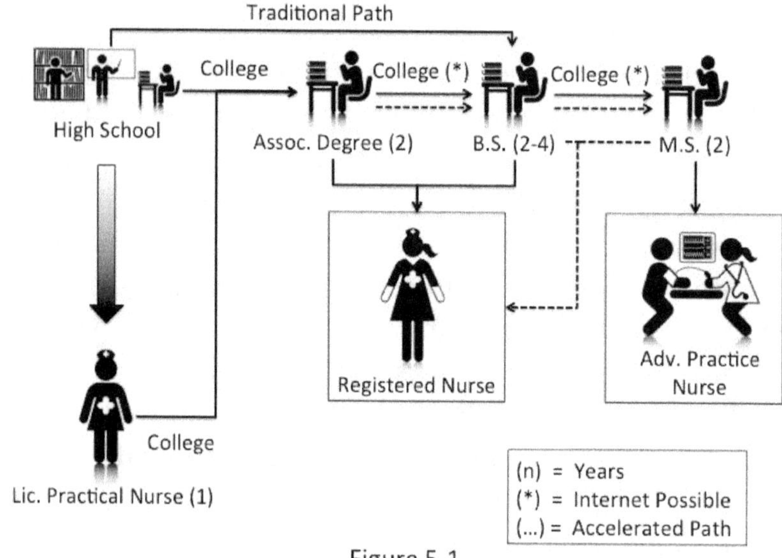

Figure 5-1
Current Model & Paths for Nursing Education

of view.

Basic nursing education begins after high school or its equivalent (Figure 5-1). The simplest path to practicing nursing is to attend a vocational or technical school for approximately one year and earn a licensed practical nursing (LPN) degree. This also requires for the individual to pass a national licensing exam developed by the National Council of State Boards of Nursing. In our country, LPNs typically provide basic bedside care, including measurement and recording of vital signs, administration of medications, monitoring of catheters and dress wounds, plus they also assist patients with grooming and mobility. Those more experienced may also supervise nursing assistants and aides. There are approximately 750,000 LPNs across the United States, with a median yearly salary that varies between $35,000 and $45,000. However, the traditional and still principal pathway for the practice of nursing is that of seeking licensing as a registered nurse (RN) (Figure 5-1). This is the type of nursing best known to the public since it is the most ubiquitous in nearly all spheres of medical care (e.g. hospital wards, intensive care units, medical clinics). In order to become an RN, the candidate must also pass a national licensing examination following the completion of a college education. Unfortunately, this is where the process becomes convoluted and less predictable because there are different ways to complete this requirement. It is conceivable for example to become an RN after just two years of college education (i.e. "associate degree" or "nursing diploma"), although the great majority of RNs have completed four years of college and have earned a baccalaureate degree. In our country, the median yearly salary for RNs varies between $65,000 and $70,000, depending on assignments, clinical environment and geography. I don't know what you think about this but I contend that this is not such a bad salary for someone who may have had only a handful of years of education following high school.

It is possible to remain an RN for a very long and fruitful career but the opportunities for advancement quickly become exhausted. Therefore, many RNs proceed to further schooling, completing a masters degree program, a step that primes them to progress to become a member of that middle management nursing class we describe in Chapter 12. The master's degree can also be the academic centerpiece of advancing to one of the various types of Advanced Practice Nurses (APN) (Table 5-1). These are individuals that acquire sufficient education to work with a greater degree of independence. Together with surgical and physician assistants, they were originally known as "Physician Extenders". Curiously, such a moniker does not seem to be as widely used as in the past, and I cannot help but have a slightly paranoid gut feeling that this trend is part of a national overreach movement for additional independence from physicians. Hold that thought... The list of different types of APNs depicted in Table 5-1 is by no means complete, and there are a variety of other programs that confer master's degrees in additional specialty role tracks, for example health systems administration, informatics, education, research management, and public health. Typically, these specialty track programs are cosponsored by nursing schools in conjunction with other disciplines, such as business or public health.

Nurse Practitioner (NP)
Adult Primary Care
Adult Acute Care
Neonatal Care
Pediatric Care
Family Primary Care
Certified Registered Nurse Anesthetist (CRNA)
Nurse Midwife (NM)
Clinical Nurse Specialist (CNS)

Table 5-1. Different types of Advanced Practice Nurses

The median yearly salary for NPs in our country approximates between $85,000 and $95,000, and that of CRNAs varies between $148,000 and $165,000. Not bad for six years of higher education! In all fairness, both NPs and CRNAs actually spend additional time as part of their education after they start their clinical practice. This type of "on the job" learning is of paramount importance in that it helps polish these individuals as true specialty professionals. Like anything else in life, however, the outcome of such a process largely depends upon two variables: the attributes of the individual himself and the quality of the environment of learning (including the supervising physician). As of the time of this writing, I have had the opportunity to work closely with a handful of NPs and my overall experience has been extremely positive. In fact, I am of the opinion that NPs *add value* to a physician's practice when optimally employed. The perfect example is the NP with whom I currently work. She and I have worked together now for about six years (longer than the standard neurology residency), and her competence in our field surpasses that of many a neurologist I know. Along these lines, I would feel perfectly confident to have her in charge of the medical care of either of my children. In my world, this is the highest compliment I can pay a medical practitioner.

However, in reviewing the nursing education process, it should be rapidly evident to the reader that there is significant heterogeneity in the making of an RN. In other words, just by looking at any RN it is impossible to be certain of what pathway has gotten him to this level. Implicitly, this also casts a shadow of a doubt as to how educated, knowledgeable and experienced the person is. The problem becomes compounded by the fact that it is now possible for some of these individuals to fulfill large portions of their educational requirements via the Internet, and web-based nursing programs continue to proliferate almost exponentially. Please understand that, in principle, I cannot possibly be critical of Internet-based education since my own business degree was acquired largely in live cyber classes. However, I submit that there is a vast difference between teaching finance or accounting using web-shared spreadsheets that can be viewed simultaneously across state lines, and teaching the skills required to be a bedside nurse. However, in the next few paragraphs it should be evident why this is being done with impunity, and how the watered-down nursing education curricula now in place lend themselves quite indulgently for such an approach.

Parenthetically, if you look closely at Figure 5–1, you may wonder why, in addition to the traditional pathways for nursing education (marked by the solid arrows), there is an alternative one (indicated by the dotted arrows). The reason is that there are individuals who achieve their nursing degrees through what is known as "accelerated" programs. These are designed to provide nursing education to those who have previously earned either baccalaureate or masters degrees in other disciplines (e.g. Bachelor of Arts). The problem with these "accelerated" programs is that they do not produce comparable professionals. Most accomplished nurses that I know frown significantly when asked about these types of curricula, and are very critical of the nurses graduating from them.

Now that we have introduced the reader to the intricacies of how convoluted (unnecessarily so in my opinion) the process of educating nurses has become, considerably different than the linear pathway of medical education (Chapter 4), let's continue by scrutinizing the intent and content of the curricula that are being offered at the present time in terms of their relevance, rationality and what I consider their *leitmotif*, one that brings to mind the changes being instituted in medical education. Just as I did when I was writing the previous chapter, I reviewed the curricula of several nursing schools, mostly local, but also others listed among the top ten in the nation.[5] The following pages represent a compilation of the most important features of their academic curricula.

I would like to begin this segment of our discussion by addressing the goals of the educational programs in nursing, as they explicitly list them in their prospectuses. Upon review of these, the first thing that catches one's attention is the use of language that is uncannily similar to the political rhetoric we hear in regards to discussions about our "healthcare system". For example, take the following sentence: *"The curriculum prepares nurses who apply theoretical and empirical knowledge from nursing, scientific, and humanistic disciplines to make evidence-based practice decisions"*. Am I reading this correctly? On the surface, it all sounds like nothing more than touchy-feely gobbledygook; however, let's dissect the content. First of all, RNs generally do not "make practice decisions", evidence-based or not. Instead, they follow the orders derived from decisions made by physicians or APNs (at least they are supposed to do so). Therefore, their knowledge of the so-called "nursing" or "scientific" disciplines can only be applied to understanding those orders. In addition, the alleged "humanistic" knowledge of nurses is rather puzzling because, in my experience, it is limited at best. Another lofty goal I found in descriptions of educational aims is that they provide graduates with the ability to *"demonstrate effective communication and collaboration skills with patients and interprofessional teams to improve healthcare outcomes"*. Interestingly, this statement could not be more inaccurate since one of the biggest problems we encounter in medicine

[5] SOURCE: U.S. News & World Report

on a daily basis is the lack of skillful communication of the nursing staff. Indeed, not one day goes by that I don't have an incident with a nurse who doesn't seem to even understand the question being asked, and often insists on responding by means of an alternative irrelevant piece of information. Another curiosity within this description is the utilization of the term "interprofessional", which frankly I had never heard. Further inquiry led me to conclude that it is a neologism introduced by the nursing community and allied health professions to designate their cronies. It is odd that nowhere in the list of program goals one reads anything about the importance of the subordinate relationship to the physicians (or APNs) who issue the orders that guide all nursing work. I cannot be persuaded that this is simply an oversight. On the contrary, leaving this topic completely out of everyone of the curricula descriptions I reviewed seems to be part of a broader agenda that gives at least impression of equal footing with physicians (I will expand on this further in Chapter 12). Finally, some of the objectives are written in plain nonsensical language. For example, *"Demonstrate the ability to independently and collaboratively apply the problem-solving process to facilitate patient, family, and community adaptation to internal and external environmental variables for the purpose of achieving maximum health"...* ...What? The more I read this statement, the more I am convinced that part of their objective is to sound important by tossing big words together into meaningless sentences, particularly since the alternative is that they are truly clueless about the realities of nursing. Wait! Now that I think about it, "clueless" may be just what they are. To further explore my original opinion, however, I ask you: What in the world is "community adaptation"? And, are they really intending to teach problem-solving techniques in college? I thought that was a subject for elementary school!

Now let's turn our attention to the actual components of the nursing school curricula. Following the first two years of college, considered "pre-nursing" and being the equivalent to five academic semesters encompassing approximately 60 credit hours total, actual nursing school includes an additional five semesters. These also comprise another 60 or so credit hours, only 23 of which (approximately one-third) involve practical clinical work. Such a design guarantees that graduates from nursing school know very little about patient care and will have to undergo an additional "bedside orientation" period of 6-12 weeks, in order to be minimally proficient in every day nursing tasks. At this point in his career, should the RN wish to continue his education by pursuing a master's degree leading to the ability to become an ANP, the next leg of the educational program varies slightly depending upon what type of ANP does the student want to become (Table 5–1). Nevertheless, the commonality between all these types of programs is that they all span five more academic semesters that comprise approximately 47 credit hours. The didactic components of these programs offer different versions of advanced classes in diagnoses, therapeutics, pharmacology, and clinical nursing. Clearly, graduates from one of these master's programs have a higher level of competence and are better prepared than those with just a baccalaureate degree. However, I still think that in looking at all these graduates, the field is not quite leveled, and what's going to determine the ultimate quality of the practitioner may well be the experienced gained after graduation. In this sense, becoming an ANP is not a lot different than the path followed by physicians, even if at a lower level of complexity.

As I embarked on researching the topic for this chapter, I came across an interesting set of dual concepts. They pertain to the availability of doctorate degrees in nursing. I did not include either of them in their main description of the path of nursing education (Figure 5–1) primarily because I think they each deserve separate consideration, the reasons for this becoming self evident in the next few paragraphs. I clearly knew the existence of a Doctor of Philosophy (PhD) in nursing prior to writing these pages. My view of it has only been confirmed by my research as a degree primarily geared at preparing nurses for careers in education, research, or both. Although earning this degree has little direct effect on the everyday practice of nursing, it undoubtedly influences it by impacting the learning process at the various levels described, as well as the decisions made by the clinical nursing "leaders" portrayed in Chapter 12 since they blindly believe and follow the publications authored by nursing PhDs (e.g. "Open Visitation" in Chapter 15).

The second form of doctorate degree I found during my research I had never encountered before. My advisors tell me that my ignorance is the result of it being created somewhat recently. Therefore, I certainly have yet to be introduced to someone who brags about being a Doctor of Nursing Practice (DNP). Following my initial awe about such an impressive title, I proceeded to carefully look at the descriptors and curriculum content, just as I did with the other degrees. It seems to me that this type of degree also steers nurses away from the bedside, more so this time into the realm of politics and policymaking. The description of one of these programs includes the following phrase: *"Graduates of the DNP program will focus on providing care to populations and communities with an emphasis on improving quality and access to underserved, diverse populations.*" I don't know about you, but I certainly do not think that such a description applies much to bedside nursing. So, what does this mean? My interpretation of the current direction nursing education is taking, beyond the baccalaureate level, is quite similar to my views on medical education changes (Chapter 4). There is an implicit paradigm change in all of these educational reforms whereby the nurses practicing at the bedside are being stripped of fundamental clinical skills for the sake of regulatory compliance, while the *nursing intelligentsia* continues to move farther and farther away from the bedside into board rooms where decisions based on pseudoscientific information and political agendas perpetuate the downgrading process of the nursing profession. Sadly, I also just learned that in the next 3-5 years, a DNP degree will be required of everyone wishing to become an NP or a CRNA.

Finally, at the risk of sounding paranoid, I must point out the alarmingly socialist tone that some of the nursing curricula descriptions seem to have taken. As a conservative, lower-case libertarian, and objectivist, it simply sent chills down my spine when I read the following passage as one of the objectives in the nursing curriculum: *"Advocate for social justice... ... policies in healthcare."* I invite you to look at the subject of "social justice" in the context of the progressive political underground movement that has been attempting to change the nature of our country along the last 100 years. I compel you to consider that there are no coincidences; that the reforms we are seeing in both medical and nursing education have taken a direction that is parallel to a totalitarian view of medical care, with the government brainwashing the future practitioners in such a way that they would become nothing but automatons that can follow regulatory guidelines without question. Curiously, this would make physicians and DNPs equivalent in the eyes of the system, making one of these groups vulnerable to be excised; but, which one of the two?

In summary, nursing education does not follow a linear path such as that displayed by medical education. Instead, there are multiple ways in which to become a bedside practicing nurse, and they're not all comparable in terms of depth of knowledge and experience. This heterogeneity translates into quality variability and an unpredictable model for the nursing profession. Current nursing programs continue to change their emphasis from educating individuals that can provide bedside care to regulation-following, policy-mongers, and glorified social workers that occupy what they call "leadership positions". The changes we have seen in nursing education mimic those of medical education, and there is a possibility that they may represent part of a bigger political agenda.

PRACTICAL DOWNGRADING

6

Polypharmacy & Psychopathology

"Any patient who takes more than five medications can have any two of them discontinued, and he will show immediate clinical improvement"

H. Houston Merritt, M.D.
Professor and Chairman of Neurology
Columbia University
(1902 - 1979)

Originally, I was going to split the information in the present chapter between two different ones. As I progressed writing both of them, it became evident to me that they belonged together. The problem of overprescribing medications in our country has epidemic proportions. There are multiple factors that contribute to this phenomenon, including educational, social, political, and practical. It appears somewhat paradoxical to me that, at a time when our country has been waging a "war on illegal drugs" for years, a more serious problem has been created with the overuse of prescription medications. In the following pages, I want to address two dimensions of this problem; two vantage points; two intertwined aspects of its *downgrading* effect; but also two potential areas of improvement in the future. The first is the propensity for an exaggerated drug prescription practice by the physician community at large. The second is the exaggerated "need" for psychoactive agents by the population served by these physicians. Together, these professional and societal tendencies spell nothing but disaster: The creation of a society of pharmacologic "zombies"! Welcome to my clinic!

Polypharmacy

It should not be surprising that following the path of Problem Oriented Medical Diagnosis (POMS) would lead to Polypharmacy. After all, for every problem there is a pill that can be prescribed regardless of the effect that the mixture of various medications can have upon the patient's health. At the time of this writing I spend most of my days discontinuing medications rather than prescribing them. In fact, not a day goes by in which I don't find myself counseling patients about the negative consequences of concurrently taking multiple medications. This type of scenario presents itself not so much because I look for it but because of the nature of my specialty. Indeed, neurologic side effects and complications from medications abound in daily practice. It is somewhat comical to be consulted to see a patient for "mental status changes" or "delirium" when, upon review of the medical record, it is blatantly evident that the patient has been receiving multiple mind-altering drugs (i.e. medications that have an effect on brain function, both intended and as a side effect). The most common offenders are opiates (i.e. narcotic painkillers), benzodiazepines (i.e. antianxiety and sedatives), psychotropics (i.e. antipsychotics and antidepressants), pain modulators (i.e. antiepileptic drugs), as well as a variety of other less frequent medications that clearly have toxic effects upon brain function. If we add to this the protean number of non-neurologic side effects produced by medications, particularly when used concurrently, the problem grows exponentially and is presently running rampant. Believe me when I say that I don't think that I can accurately portray in these pages the enormity of the situation, but I will do my best to show the reader how this subject must be brought to the front of our discussion of the quality of medical care, as well as the downgrading effect of our current practices. In order to illustrate the issue, I randomly chose one week of my practice and reviewed the medication lists of all of the patients seen in clinic, with particular attention to the number and classes of drugs simultaneously being taken. I then probed the data using the simplest of techniques. The results are displayed in Table 6-1.

A cursory review of my findings from this small retrospective analysis shows the magnitude of the problem we are addressing. The patients whose records were reviewed averaged *six concurrent medications*, with 10 of them (14%) taking 10 or more drugs. Can you even imagine having to take 10 (some up to 15 or 24) different prescription medications on a daily basis? It's a full time job! What else can you possibly do with your time? What do you think the chances of having side effects from these are? In my experience, it is often difficult to comply with taking a single antibiotic for two weeks! Parenthetically, you may think that looking at one week of my practice is not representative of reality. I assure you that it is! In fact, I would argue that my analysis is rather conservative since that particular week we had 10 (14%) patients under the age of 18 because we still see a fair number of minors in our practice (The next available appointment for any child or teenager at the Pediatric Neurology clinic in Birmingham's Children's Hospital is over six months away!). In general, minors do not have such a long lifetime and, therefore, have not had the opportunity to be exposed to as many medications as adults. That said, they constitute a special problem, not because of the number of medications given to them but because of the types. I will address this topic later in the chapter since their issue is more pertinent to the widespread prevalence of psychopathology in our society. In this context, I will also address not only the quantity of the medications given to minors, but their types as they pertain to the so-called "mental illness".

Population	
Number of Patients (Male/Female))	73 (31/42)
Ages (Years)	9 - 88 (Mean = 51)
Medication Profiles	
Total Medications per Patient	0 – 24 (Mean = 6)
Ingestion of Mind-Altering Drugs	
Patients Taking Opiates (Pain Narcotics)	13 (18%)
Patients Taking Benzodiazepines (Tranquilizers)	9 (12%)
Patients Taking Antidepressants	22 (30%)
Patients Taking Hypnotics (Sleeping Aids)	9 (12%)
Patients Taking Amphetamines (Stimulants)	2 (3%)
Concurrent Ingestion of Mind-Altering Drugs	
Total Patients Taking at Least One	36 (49%)
Total Patients Taking at Least Two	20 (27%)
Total Patients Taking at Least Three	9 (12%)

Table 6-1. Profile of One Week of Patient Medications

Continuing our discussion, however, I would like to reiterate my position regarding the principal role of the physician being that of *promoting patients' quality of life, rather than maintaining their heart beating indefinitely and despite the cost of doing so.* Therefore, prescribing medications just because they "solve" a problem, while ignoring the resulting undesirable side effects that negatively affect quality of life is not at all reasonable. The disturbing practices that lead to Polypharmacy breach certain fundamental principles of clinical therapeutics, most importantly: 1) The importance of introducing new medications one at a time, and 2) The soundness of introducing any medication at the smallest possible dose. I witness violations of these principles on a daily basis, supporting my contention that we have a serious problem with the inclusion of logic in medical education. Let's expand on each one of these two problems some more.

In general, there are powerful reasons not to initiate more than one medication at a time. The most important of these is *decreased predictability*. It is impossible to know how two medications that a patient has never taken before will interact in terms of absorption, effectiveness, and side effect profile. For each one of these therapeutic phases, the relationship between any two drugs can be analyzed following a somewhat algebraic pattern: They either have an *additive* (i.e. they increase the effect and/or side effects of each other), a *neutral* (i.e. they have no effect on each other and act as they would independently) or a *canceling* (i.e. they counteract each other) effect. There is also the possibility of a mixed interaction (Figure 6-1). For example, two medications may cancel each other's intended beneficial effect, while adding to each other's side effects. Thus, even though those who simultaneously prescribe more than one drug are banking on achieving a neutral effect, this is actually the least common outcome from our point of view. Typically, the patients experience difficulties relative to lessened effectiveness, augmented side effects, or both. This problem is particularly prominent due to the widespread utilization of mind-altering drugs. Please consider that in our informal review, almost half (49%) of the patients were being given at least one of these medications, and 12% were ingesting *three or more at a time!* Shocked? It gets worse; I purposely did not

		BENEFITS		
		CANCELING	NEUTRAL	ADDITIVE
SIDE EFFECTS	CANCELING	BAD	POSITIVE	POSITIVE
	NEUTRAL	BAD	POSITIVE	POSITIVE
	ADDITIVE	BAD	BAD	NEUTRAL

Figure 6-1
Potential Algebraic Interaction of Any Two Medications

include in my assessment of this problem the use of medications to prevent seizures and headaches, which 38% of the patients were being prescribed, and all of which can alter brain function. My reason for excluding them is that in any Neurology clinic this class of medications is expected and common and, therefore, its frequent utilization would bias the results. Thus, this supports my previous statement that, if anything, my analysis is probably erring on the conservative side.

The second principle that is commonly forgone in daily practice is that of initiating medications at the lowest dose possible. Does this not make sense to you? Why would I want to give you 50mg of *any drug*, if 10mg can achieve the desired effect? Well, it is done daily and usually because someone reads a published study in which the larger dose was found to be the "most effective". I want to refer the reader back to Chapter 2 and the problems we identified with studies that lead to Evidence-Based Medicine (EBM). The commonest example of this problem is the drug Lipitor®, used to treat cholesterol problems and widely advertised in national television. The minimum dose available is 10mg but yet it is commonly introduced to patients in doses of 40-80mg because these doses have been found to be the most effective. Curiously, the practitioners that follow this strategy, who stand tall and praise the necessity of practicing EBM do not realize that Epidemiology and Public Health (i.e. the collective treatment of our population) are not clinical medicine (i.e. the individualized treatment of each patient), and clearly have not pondered about the second pillar of EBM: The *clinical expertise* necessary to apply the existing knowledge to each clinical situation, and for which there is no substitute (Chapter2). Needless to say, the number of individuals with early side effects from Lipitor® is significant and the problem has been recently compounded since a generic version of the drug (i.e. Atorvastatin) is now available (see Chapter 21).

There are other contributing factors to the dissemination of Polypharmacy. For example, in Chapter 3 we discussed *"The Multi-doctor Gambit"* and referred to its implications. Well, guess what? One of the consequences of this practice is staring us right in the face: *Multiple physicians with prescription pads not paying attention to what each other is doing!* The truth is that it is easy to be so involved in the "problem" assigned to one's specialty from the patient's master list, that one does not take into consideration the rest of the patient's issues, and the medications being given for those. Moreover, the patients are often complicit since they generally fail to keep track of their medications so they can keep every physician accurately informed of what they are taking. This is not a small problem, I assure you. In our clinic for example, every patient is given the opportunity at check in to review the list of medications we have on record, edit it and sign off (we actually get their signature) on it. However, the failure rate for this task being completed accurately approximates 75-80%! Moreover, patients almost never bring their pills bottles to clinic as they are repeatedly instructed to do. This, in my view, is another sign of a culture of entitlement, in which patient's *rights* abound but patient's *responsibilities* are willfully neglected (Chapter 18). Still, and in all fairness, the overwhelming majority of patients with whom I discuss reducing their list of medications are eager to make such changes because they find it burdensome to take so many pills. The minority typically includes patients that we will discuss in the second half of this chapter.

At this point in our discussion it is fair to ask: What motivates this type of prescription habits on the part of physicians? The root cause of this problem, at least in my opinion, is a combination of *insufficient knowledge of pharmacology* and *intellectual laziness.* In Chapter 4 we outlined the significant changes that have been introduced during the last 30 years in medical education. As you may recall, one of the motivating factors for the current medical school curricula to include more clinical experience in the first two years, instead of the traditional emphasis on basic sciences (including Pharmacology), was the medical students perception that the information was not going to be that useful in their ultimate practice. This has become a self-fulfilling prophecy and the current medical graduates have substantial knowledge deficits regarding drugs and their proper clinical utilization. However, since they never thought they were going to need such information, they don't miss it! As a result, physicians of the recent generations prescribe from the hip, as part of a reflexive behavior modeled after guidelines and triggered by entries in problem lists. Moreover, as new medications become available in the market, any additional pharmacology education is acquired via the ubiquitous pharmaceutical sales representatives whose visits are embedded with pseudoscientific platitudes about how superior the medication they represent is in comparison to the competition. This paradigm explains why nearly every patient who complains of burning pain is currently being treated with gabapentin, regardless of the cause.

Finally, intellectual laziness is that pervasive characteristic that makes physicians choose the easier path of submission instead of that of obsessive self reliance in the face of medical diagnostic and therapeutic challenges. Let's face it; it is much easier to follow guidelines than to make independent decisions regarding the best clinical course of action for any given scenario. It is also easier to loot from the offered solutions than to create your own by means of independent study and personal research. It is a safer position, more defensible in the event of any peer inquiry (the peers of course being part of the Kool-Aid® drinking followers, who worship and blindly submit to the *medical intelligentsia*), and devoid of any inkling of innovation. The corollary of embracing intellectual laziness is that it creates a responsibility vacuum; and we all know how much nature abhors such a thing. Thus, when physicians become intellectual followers instead of leaders, the vacuum created will be filled by pharmacists or will lead to the proliferation of local regulatory bodies (e.g. "Pharmacy and Therapeutics Committees"). Once again, the collective progressively controls the individuals and force its agenda into the clinical environment. Unfortunately, the downgraded practice of overprescribing does not exist without a complementary counterpart behavior on the patient's side of the equation.

Psychopathology

Everyone wants a pill and, guess what? Everyone else in healthcare is willing to prescribe one. These two statements summarize a major aspect of the present status of clinical medicine in our country. In discussing the subject with nearly every experienced practicing colleague, there is almost complete consensus that the amount of psychopathology we come in contact in everyday practice is not only large, but it continues to grow daily. Such a conclusion is independent of the specialty or the experience of the person discussing it. How is this possible? Why is it taking place? What is its impact? These questions should be openly discussed because of the ramifications of such a large proportion of our fellow citizens either displaying symptoms of psychopathology, or simply being treated with psychopharmacologic agents that have become ubiquitous to our daily existence. How big is this problem? Well, let's look back at Table 6-1. As we mentioned earlier, almost half (49%) of the patients in our review were taking at least one mind-altering drug, and 12% were ingesting three or more at a time. What types of drugs are these? I included in my review opiates (i.e. pain killing narcotics), benzodiazepines (i.e. tranquilizers), antidepressants, hypnotics (i.e. sleeping aids) and amphetamines (i.e. stimulants). This pattern of drugs means that, at least in the small sample of my patients, about 30% carry a diagnosis of depression and about 13% a diagnosis of anxiety. Another 13% apparently has insomnia, which is an interesting finding since this is a common symptom of the former two. Do we really believe that one out of every three members of our society suffers from depression? I assure you, they believe they do! However, think about it; this means that the prevalence of depression has the magnitude of a pandemic. Does this make sense? Stay tuned for an alternative explanation.

It is important to recognize that there is a difference between *bona fide* mental illness and the topic of this chapter. Let me clarify the difference between the two. Mental illness, that which includes conditions such as bipolar disorder and schizophrenia, usually results from an inherent defect in neurotransmitter physiology. These neurotransmitters are brain chemical compounds that allow signaling within specific neural networks. Either a deficiency or an excess of neurotransmitters give rise to dysfunction of the network involved, which is translated into symptoms. For example, a deficiency of the neurotransmitter dopamine results in a condition known as Parkinson's disease. Similarly, the term *mental illness* refers to a range of neurochemical disorders that require pharmacologic manipulation in order to bring balance to brain function. These conditions are not the result of external factors or a behavioral response to the daily challenges that life presents us along the way. They do not include situations such as *"I feel depressed because my girlfriend dumped me!"* and they cannot be equated with the results of our personal circumstances, no matter how miserable we may feel. As such, they generally cannot be prevented and require expert help (i.e. psychologists and psychiatrists) for the patients to maintain their quality of life.

Conversely, what I mean by psychopathology is a different category of conditions, largely those that represent a behavioral answer to a stimulus originated as part of life. This is not to say that all patients with psychopathology are unworthy of pharmacologic intervention or expert treatment. Take for example the diagnosis of posttraumatic stress disorder (PTSD). These patients have legitimate problems derived from having been exposed to stressful conditions that sometimes are unimaginable by the rest of us. Lives can be shattered by rape, attempted murder, war, or any one of various negative experiences that leave behind a destructive set of memories. Even if this is the case, however, it must be clear that pharmacologic intervention leads to an imbalance of neurotransmitter physiology (i.e. the medications are liable to result in that increase or decrease of certain transmitters whose levels were within the normal range prior to treatment), and that expert treatment must also include non-pharmacologic intervention (e.g. counseling). Furthermore, this is an area of medicine in which we cannot overemphasize the danger of just throwing pills at the patient, particularly when we consider the significant side effects of the medications typically used. The problem that I would like to discuss in this second half of the chapter, however, is that relative to the question "Where do we draw the line?"

Indeed, the psychopathology that I refer to in our discussion constitutes a simpler and more widespread problem; a problem whose origins can be traced to the interaction between life's unhappiness and our response to it. A glimpse of this problem can be easily seen throughout our discussions of medical education (Chapter 4), medical emergencies (Chapter 16), the obsession with pain (Chapter 17) and the culture of entitlement (Chapter 18). Moreover, the socioeconomic situation of our country contributes to this problem by providing a perfect cradle for this type of infirmities to sprout out of the unhappiness of people in general. The latter may be the consequence of wrong personal choices, faulty upbringing, or simply bad luck. In any case, however, the result is almost identical: *Hordes of people seeking and being prescribed psychoactive (i.e. mind-altering) drugs by the handful!*

As we have seen in the previous pages, this phenomenon of medical practice translates into a large proportion of patients seen across our nation carrying some type of psychiatric diagnosis, the most common offenders being "anxiety", "depression" and "bipolar disorder". It further translates into every one of these individuals taking one and, frequently, multiple psychoactive drugs (Table 6-1); it is also common for these patients to concurrently take narcotic painkillers (i.e. opiates), complicating the side effect unpredictability of the mixture. The culture of the use of opiates will be further discussed in Chapter 17. Interestingly, and although it would seem intuitive that my point of view is artificially biased due to the overlapping nature of neurology and psychiatry, everyday discussions with many physicians has led me to conclude that the problem is widespread and quite uniform across medicine. The profile of the typical patient is not difficult to recognize: *An unhappy individual with erratic ill-defined complaints or greatly magnified simple problems, overmedicated and with clear signs of medication dependence (either physical, psychological or both).*

The consequences of patients fitting this profile are plenty, and they insinuate themselves through every aspect of healthcare, leading to its downgrading. These patients are more likely to complain endlessly, to respond poorly to any treatment provided, and to constantly shift their priorities from real medical issues to unimportant nuisances that represent excuses for how unhappy their personal lives are. They crave attention and they demand medications, irrespective of whether they work or not. Most of us in medical practice dread finding ourselves in an exam room with one of these patients. It is as unproductive as trying to hold gelatin between one's fingers; their behavior resulting in long-drawn-out clinical encounters and the obligatory additional testing required for one of two reasons: Either because we often have to give these patients the benefit of the doubt (remember the old saying *"Even crazy people have to die of something"*), or because it is the only way to satisfy the anxiety that drives these individuals to repeatedly (or rather endlessly) insist that *"Something must be wrong!"* or that *"Something has to be done!"*. Personally, I find the experience of dealing with this type of patient exhausting and I have compared it to the characteristic life-draining effect exerted by the *Dementors* of the *Harry Potter* series on anyone they encounter. Nevertheless, it is becoming increasingly frequent that all of us are placed in a position to have to deal with this problem. Here lies the dilemma: *How can we truly help these very difficult patients?*

Perhaps the answer must include a large dose of introspection and a sense of fairness. As with many of the important decisions we face in life, the answer is in the mirror! We must face the fact that the propagation of this phenomenon across our population could not have been possible without the complicit participation of physicians who are unwilling to look at patients in the eye and tell them the truth: That the bulk of their complaints have an underlying psychological basis; that they do not need an excessive amount of psychoactive medications; that they might be better off subjecting themselves to psychotherapy. Instead, the easy path is to put pharmacologic Band-Aids® on the "problems" and move on! The fact is that we can be more dangerous with a prescription pad than with a scalpel, and until we are willing to recognize this danger, we will continue to perpetuate these patients' situation to the detriment of their overall well being. In my experience (I seem to find myself delivering these news to patients almost daily), it is very difficult not only to be truthful and factual, but also to withstand the typical response to such sobering statements. Patients and families do not want to agree with or believe what they are being told. They cling to their previously-given, or the internet-searched diagnoses with ferocity. I certainly do not envy the psychiatrists to whom I refer these patients after I have had a heart-to-heart discussion with them. Unfortunately, just like alcohol and drug addiction, unless the patient is ready to be delivered from his demons, no one can accomplish this for him.

Since most of us in practice agree that this is a more prevalent problem than it used to be, it begs the question: *why is it so?* I cannot imagine that over the last three decades this problem has become more visible because we used to miss its presence in the past. This would mean that several generations of physicians have failed to recognize many of these patients across the nation and not just in one community. The likelihood of such an explanation is simply infinitesimally small and akin to justifying the present existence of dubious diagnoses such as *Fibromyalgia*. Conversely, it seems much more likely that these diagnoses are somewhat artificial, used as crutches or excuses that entitle the patients to justify their need for more pills. In my opinion, psychopathology is strictly the product of the progressive psychosocial breakdown experienced by our society, with weakening of the family unit, exposure to countless daily stressors, reprioritization of personal goals, and the development of wrongful expectations and entitlements. In any case, right or wrong, the answer is not the indiscriminate utilization of mind-altering drugs.

In summary, polypharmacy predictably accompanied the introduction of POMD as a reflexive therapeutic phenomenon that matches each "problem" to a drug intended to solve it. The use of multiple medications is a frequent practice in our country and the consequences include an enhanced production of side effects, particularly when mind-altering drugs are being used. The factors that underscore the practice of polypharmacy include ignorance of pharmacology and intellectual laziness by physicians. In parallel, the prevalence of psychopathology in medical practice continues to grow. This appears to be different than mental illness in the strict sense, and most likely results from a variety of psychosocial issues. However, physicians need to understand their role in worsening and perpetuating this serious problem, so they can be part of the solution. Honesty in our interaction with these patients, unpleasant as it may be, carries with a component of fairness upon it is possible to build real solutions without needing to resort to the indiscriminate prescription of drugs.

7

Physician Compensation

"In a higher phase of a communist society, after the enslaving subordination of the individual to the division of labor, and therewith also the antithesis between mental and physical labor, has vanished... ...only then can the narrow horizon of bourgeois right be crossed in its entirety and Society inscribed on its banners: From each according to his ability, and to each according to his needs"

Karl Marx
German Philosopher, Economist, and Revolutionary Socialist
(1818 - 1883)

The great majority of physicians I know did not endeavor to practice medicine for the primary purpose of making obscene amounts of money. In fact, truth be told, there are presently numerous ways in which one can make a much better living without as much commitment, sacrifice and pain. Nevertheless, one of the most widespread forms of class warfare in our society, even though it is hardly ever mentioned in public, is being waged against physicians. This war has been instigated by the government, fueled by all third party payers, and ideologically supported by a large portion of our population. At the center of this feud is the commonly held idea that all physicians are filthy rich, live in colossal mansions, drive expensive European cars, and regularly take lavish vacations. Nowhere in the sophistry that pervades the arguments made for increasing regulation of physicians' incomes does one see factored the enormous investment we have made in terms of personal time, family time, energy, and finances (let's not forget those student loans). It is, in fact, easier for our society to accept that Peyton Manning recently signed a contract with the Denver Broncos for $95 million over a few years, than understand that a physician would want to earn several extra thousand dollars a year by lecturing, consulting, or moonlighting. The former is called talented and successful, while the latter is simply referred to as *greedy*. I beg the reader's indulgence; it is not that I think Mr. Manning is not worth such contract (let's not forget that I am a University of Tennessee alumnus). On the contrary, as a firm supporter of the free market system, as long as there is demand for his talent, I think he should be able to earn as much as anyone is willing to pay him. The issue I am raising by making the previous comparison is that of the double standard embraced by a society that has its priorities markedly mixed up. Thus, the resentment commonly engendered by the topic of physicians' incomes represents a combination of social envy and ignorance of the subject at hand. In the next few pages I will examine the current status of physician's compensation and how it compares amid various other societal groups. I will also put in perspective how the system is engineered to consistently devalue our profession at the expense of bureaucratic control and crony profitability. Finally, I will impress upon the reader a concept that is almost never heard in the political rhetoric of either side of the aisle: *Medicine in the United States is already socialized!*

That last statement may have caught a few by surprise. What do I mean by that? How is it possible? It is actually very simple. The "inconvenient truth" regarding physician compensation, one that has been operating for decades now, is that it does not matter how much physicians think their work is worth; they will get paid whatever the government dictates. In other words, no matter how much a physician bills for his services, the payment is going to be discounted based on reimbursement formulas that originate with the government [i.e. Center for Medicare and Medicaid Services (CMS)], and which are quickly mimicked by all other payers. Nonetheless, when is the last time you heard this topic discussed in national television? How about never? Still, I invite you to remember this point the next time someone engages in an exchange about the "business" of medicine. The "business" of medicine... What a farce! If medicine is truly a "business", how is it that the buyer sets the price of the product, and does so by force? When have you ever gone to Sears or Macy's and, once at the checkout counter, have you told the clerk that you were going to pay only 60% of what the total of your purchase was? Moreover, could you have followed such statement with the assertion that the store had no recourse but to accept by force the discount you were imposing? Well, this is exactly what we are told on a daily basis by CMS and its cronies. Sounds fascistic, doesn't it? The truth is that the so-called "business" of medicine is a hoax because the current model is like no business in any free market. In fact, as we will see below, the price fixing that characterizes our healthcare system is precisely the antithesis of the free market, and as such, a significant feature of the financial meltdown we have witnessed in our profession. Along these lines, and paraphrasing Fredrick Hayek, the centralized system of medical compensation we currently have in our country is nothing but a *road to medical serfdom*. It does not experience any of the beneficial effects of supply and demand, or the self-regulating effect of a price-based system. Furthermore, as I will show below, it continues to grow in the predictable bureaucratic frenzy that accompanies the ever-expanding government control of healthcare.

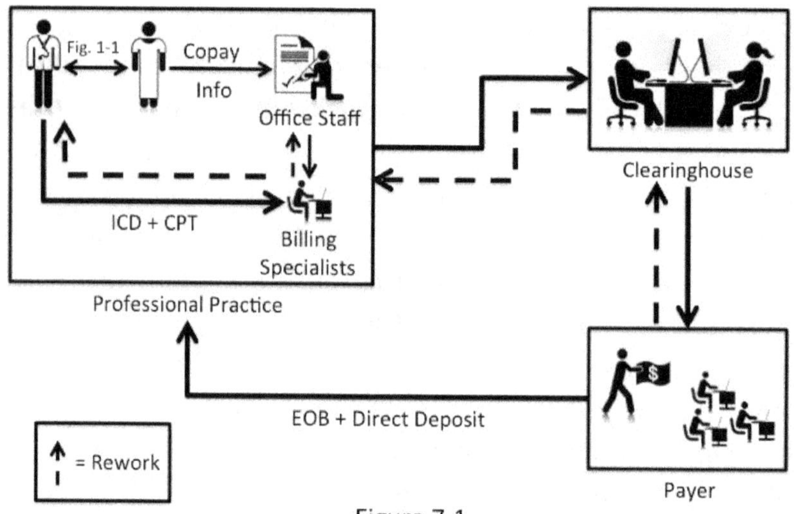

Figure 7-1
The Process of Professional Billing & Reimbursement
(See Text for Explanation)

The downgrading effect of the current physician compensation culture is compounded further because physicians' payments are not only discounted without any recourse, but the mechanism (the only mechanism!) available to bill and to get paid for services is so convoluted that it represents more of an obstacle to payment than a *bona fide* compensation tool (Figure 7-1). At a time when anyone can buy a car or a house in the Internet with a simple click of the mouse, and consummate the transaction securely, processing a medical insurance claim is a painstaking, inefficient, redundant and impractical system. I want to walk the reader through this process, while pointing out details that illustrate how it does nothing but contribute to the downgrading of the healthcare system. First of all, it is important that we point out that physicians do not get "paid", they get "reimbursed". This difference underscores how punitive the system is when it comes with physician compensation.

Let's begin by examining how the government reimbursement formula works since it will help understand the rest of the process. All activities physicians carry out, whether a patient encounter (e.g. a clinic visit), a diagnostic test (e.g. colonoscopy) or a therapeutic intervention (e.g. removal of the appendix), are altogether referred to as *procedures* and each is assigned an identifying code; an exclusive five digit number that differentiates them from the rest. These codes were created by the American medical Association (AMA), who holds the intellectual property rights (a point worth remembering for future reference in some of our discussions), and are all assembled as the Current Procedural Terminology (CPT). These CPT codes are developed by a 17 member committee known as the CPT Editorial Panel, which includes 11 members appointed by the AMA, and the rest by the Blue Cross/Blue Shield (BC/BS) Association, the American Hospital Association (AHA), the Health Insurance Association of America and, or course, CMS. These CPT codes MUST be used for billing and, in order for payment to be approved, they MUST be linked to the appropriate International Classification of Diseases (ICD) code. The theory is that each CPT code can only be justified (and paid) for patients with the appropriate diagnoses. Reasonable? On the surface but, wait, there is more! In addition to CPT codes, of which there are approximately 7,000, billing often requires the addition of modifiers that indicate circumstances that will alter the reimbursement. For example, attaching modifier "-50" indicates that the procedure being billed was *bilateral*. Imagine the countless opportunities for error that exist when we are required to choose, from thousands of possible ones, the only codes and modifiers combination that will lead to payment for each clinical situation. Such errors, when plotted into the process depicted in Figure 7-1 can only lead to rework, waste, payment delays, and... ...Oh yes, increased *indirect cost* of healthcare. The latter is a concept that I will cover throughout the book since it is something not quite addressed by the public discourse of either political party.

So, now that we have introduced the concept of coding, let's examine how CMS determines the amount to be paid for each CPT code. This is where it begins to get noteworthy so hold on! Before 1985, payments to physicians were made according to the so-called *Usual, Customary and Reasonable* (UCR) scheme. The UCR was originally part of the Social Security Act of 1965, but it met with criticisms of unfairness at both ends. Claims were made that UCR undervalued clinical activities and overvalued surgical ones, creating a degree of unfairness among the physician community. Mind you that, despite its name and its appearance on the surface, UCR still dictated payments without discriminating between practitioners but rather homogeneously, effectively treating medical practice as a commodity (see below). More recently, President Bush (41) signed the Omnibus Budget Reconciliation Act of 1989 and, with it, he switched CMS to the current Resource-Based Relative Value Scale (RBRVS) system of payment that has been in effect since 1992. As we will see, this had the effect of a steroid injection into the complexity of the system, and led to ominous economic consequences.

The RBRVS assigns each physician activity (i.e. each CPT code) a relative value which is adjusted by geographic region using the Geographic Pricing Cost Index (GPCI). The relative value of each CPT code is expressed as Relative Value Units (RVU). In addition, the final payments are calculated by considering three factors: the physician work in RVUs (52%), the practice expense (PE = 44%) and the malpractice expense (MP = 4%), all of which are then multiplied by a conversion factor (CF) determined annually by CMS (the CY 2012 conversion factor is $34.0376). The final formula looks like this:

*[(CPT RVU * GPCI) + (PE RVU *PE GPCI) + (MP RVU * MP GPCI)] * CF*

The responsibility to develop and revise RVUs falls on the Specialty Society Relative Value Scale Update Committee (known as RUC). This is a 29-member committee that meets privately (anyone attending signs a confidentiality agreement and no one external to the RUC is allowed to know the particulars of their meetings) three times per year to discuss RVUs and advise CMS on changes. The committee includes 23 members from different specialty societies, plus two members appointed by the AMA (One of them the Chair), and representatives from the CPT Editorial Panel, the American Osteopathic Association (AOA), the Health Care Professions Advisory Committee and the Practice Expense Review Committee. It should be immediately apparent to the reader that a system organized this way is nothing but a price fixing scheme; a cartel that represents the exact opposite of the free market system, and carries with it all types of historically predictable negative consequences. The most important of these is recognized by anyone with a working knowledge of economics. In a free market, prices rise because the amount demanded exceeds the supply *at the existing prices*, and they fall due to the opposite scenario. The former is referred to as a *"shortage"* and the latter as a *"surplus"*. Based upon these concepts, it should have been easy to predict that one of the effects of the RVU compensation fixing on medical care is analogous to that of rent control on housing, an artificial and self-perpetuating shortage!

As I illustrate in Figure 7-1, however, the process of billing and reimbursement for physician services begins when the patient shows up to any professional practice and provides the office staff with two things: Information and a co-pay. The former must comprise details about his healthcare insurance, particularly the carrier and the policy. All of this information must be verified by the office staff and flawlessly entered into the electronic system used for billing, otherwise the system will reject the claim at one of the subsequent points described below, sometimes simply because one digit is incorrect. The office staff must also record the collection of the co-pay since the claim may not be paid unless the patient has contributed this required amount, or worse, it may be considered fraud! How much is this co-pay? It varies widely; Medicare patients pay 20% of services after they have met their $140 annual deductible, while Medicaid patients are required to pay $1. As I will mention in Chapter 18, it is not unusual for us to have significant difficulties collecting this co-pay, especially from groups with a significant entitlement mentality. From the economic point of view, the co-pay gives the patient a false image of the *total price* of the service being provided, and therefore is a source of misinformation. This compounds the negative effects of price control described earlier, but also underscores the fundamental economic flaws in the system, and possibly the most important avenue for future solutions.

Once the patient has been seen, the physician chooses the appropriate ICD and CPT codes for the encounter and gives this information to a billing specialist (either in-house or outsourced) who reviews it and, once he determines it is satisfactory, transmits it in encrypted form to a clearinghouse. In turn, the clearinghouse *scrubs* (checks it for errors) the claim and transmits it to the insurance carrier in an encrypted electronic form. Then, the claim is either accepted or rejected and, if accepted, reimbursement is made by direct deposit. In either case, the clearinghouse and the practice are notified of the decision of the carrier via an Explanation of Benefits (EOB) communication. Notice the unnecessary complexity and redundancy of this system, as well as the numerous opportunities for error. Let's cover in more detail the steps described, beginning with the physician's responsibility of choosing the correct ICD and CPT codes, at the risk of being audited and charged with fraud, particularly by CMS.

Choosing the ICD and CPT codes correctly may seem like an easy task for a physician to carry out, especially one with extensive clinical experience. You would be sadly mistaken to take this step for granted since the choices to be made have nothing to do with clinical medicine. Rather, they are another example of the games engineered by government employees and their stooges as hurdles that interpose themselves between physicians and their livelihood. Games that are played by rules that obey no logic, and that change nearly every year, making billing proficiency an almost impossibility. Don't believe me? Let's look at the ICD codes available for a very common diagnosis in my specialty:

Migraine (Table 7-1). As you can see, it is not sufficient to make a proper diagnosis. One has to specify all sorts of details that, frankly, are clinically irrelevant and should not alter treatment in any way. Surprised? Wait! There is more; I only included in Table 7-1 the three most common categories of migraine codes for the sake of brevity. In reality, there are another seven categories (346.3 through 346.9) of migraine codes, each with four subcategories. Personally, of the 40 possible five digit ICD codes for migraine, I typically use only four of them. In addition, I have had to change their description to more clinically meaningful ones than those shown in Table 7-1 and which are the defaults in every electronic medical record (EMR) software; as certified by government.

346.00 Migraine with aura, without mention of intractable migraine without mention of status migrainosus

346.01 Migraine with aura, with intractable migraine, so stated, without mention of status migrainosus

346.02 Migraine with aura, without mention of intractable migraine with status migrainosus

346.03 Migraine with aura, with intractable migraine, so stated, with status migrainosus

346.10 Migraine without aura, without mention of intractable migraine without mention of status migrainosus

346.11 Migraine without aura, with intractable migraine, so stated, without mention of status migrainosus

346.12 Migraine without aura, without mention of intractable migraine with status migrainosus

346.13 Migraine without aura, with intractable migraine, so stated, with status migrainosus

346.20 Variants of migraine, not elsewhere classified, without mention of intractable migraine, without mention of status migrainosus

346.21 Variants of migraine, not elsewhere classified, with intractable migraine, so stated, without mention of status migrainosus

346.22 Variants of migraine, not elsewhere classified, without mention of intractable migraine with status migrainosus

346.23 Variants of migraine, not elsewhere classified, with intractable migraine, so stated, with status migrainosus

Table 7-1. ICD for Patients with Migraine

Now let's turn our attention to the physician's task of choosing the CPT codes. Ah! What worthless energy expenditure! The CPT codes available to bill for patient encounters, also known as the Evaluation & Management (E/M) codes, have been organized based upon the complexity of the history, the complexity of the examination, and the complexity of the decision making process; in addition, they are assigned a presumptive physician face-to-face time with the patient (Table 7-2). Interestingly, the definitions for each of these criteria (except of course time) are written in such a way as to make compliance difficult and auditing easy. The obsession with objectivizing everything has led to a variety of consequences, including the development of Electronic Medical records (EMR) software that can calculate the appropriate CPT code from data entered for each encountered. The result, as we will discuss in Chapters 14 and 23, has been that electronic medical records read more like invoices than like clinically useful notes. The disincentive, particularly for the intellectually lazy, is simple to understand: *"Why should I waste time in making notes that are clinically meaningful, so long as my notes get my work reimbursed?"* and, *"Let whoever is reading my note figure out what it actually says!"* In fact, this is what we see everyday, clinical notes that meet all components for the highest level of billing, but whose content is largely useless. I will present examples in Chapters 14 and 23, when we address the topic of *"Meaningful Use"*.

Code	History	Examination	Decision	Face-to Face
99201	Prob. Focused	Prob. Focused	Straightforward	10 min
99202	Prob. Expanded	Prob. Expanded	Straightforward	20 min
99203	Detailed	Detailed	Low Complexity	30 min
99304	Comp.	Comp.	Mod. Complexity	45 min
99205	Comp.	Comp.	High Complexity	60 min

Table 7-2. CPT codes for New Outpatient Visits

Specialty	Average	Median	Median RVUs	Comp. / RVU
Int. Medicine	$193,581	$191,198	4,691	$41.73
Hospitalists	$200,602	$210,250	3,810	$54.09
OBGYN	$258,363	$285,812	6,750	$43.90
Surgery	$321,955	$320,116	6,893	$49.25
Pediatrics	$179,291	$186,641	4,927	$38.44
Neurology	$228,871	$234,505	4,915	$49.11

Table 7-3 (See Text for Explanation)

So how much money do physicians make? Undoubtedly, there are exceptional specialties whose compensation is very significant, some even into the seven figures per year (Neurosurgery and Orthopedic Surgery come to mind). However, the overwhelming majority of us have to hump it for living. I have itemized general figures about physician compensation in Table 7-3. The examples I chose include the four major general specialties [Medicine, Surgery, Pediatrics, and Obstetrics-Gynecology (OBGYN)], as well as Hospital Medicine, which is a popular offshoot of Internal Medicine. Finally, I added my own specialty (i.e. Neurology) for perspective. The first column represents the fair market value of compensation averaged across five surveys conducted between 2009 and 2011 by different firms. The three remaining columns display the median of physician annual compensation (in 2009 dollars), the median of annual RVUs, and the median of annual compensation/RVUs ratio [Data collected by the Medical Group Management Association (MGMA)]. As you can see, the bulk of physicians can be grouped around the $250,000 earning level. I guess that places us within the so-called *middle class* that I hear so much in the political news nowadays. It certainly does not place us among the *very rich*

that our current administration wants to tax further so they pay their "fair share"; whatever that means...
For comparison purposes, consider that the median salary for attorneys is $144,720, while the following medians apply to various other professions: Chief Executive Officer (CEO) = $728,399, Chief Operating Officer (COO) = $444,873, Dentist = $142,090, Veterinarian = $94,409, Engineers = $80,517, Accountants = $64,394. I have left out the compensation of professional athletes and movie stars due to the obvious difficulties in making fair comparisons. However, although at first glance our take-home pay may seem quite competitive, I ask the reader to please consider the years of education required (see Chapter 4), the hours we work, the convoluted system required for billing and payment described, the effect of discounted fees on the clinical volume necessary to make a living, the exaggerated expenditures in professional fees and malpractice insurance premiums (see Chapter 9), and the limitations in entrepreneurship created by government regulations (see Chapter 8). The other professions listed can hardly compare in any of these categories.

Code	Type	CMS	BC/BS	Alacaid
99201	New Outpatient	$38.40	$37.00	$30.00
99202	New Outpatient	$66.55	$49.00	$53.00
99203	New Outpatient	$69.32	$73.00	$78.00
99304	New Outpatient	$147.99	$104.00	$111.00
99205	New Outpatient	$152.30	$155.00	$142.00
99211	Est. Outpatient	$17.94	$26.00	$17.00
99212	Est. Outpatient	$38.80	$39.00	$31.00
99213	Est. Outpatient	$64.93	$62.75	$42.00
99214	Est. Outpatient	$96.30	$95.00	$67.00
99215	Est. Outpatient	$129.66	$122.00	$98.00

Table 7-4. Current Reimbursement by CPT Codes

How do we make this money? Just the same way as porcupines mate: *Very carefully!* As noted earlier, each CPT code has an assigned reimbursement rate, both by CMS and the other carriers. If a claim is paid, the typical reimbursement rates are predetermined and exemplified in Table 7-4. I have included the rates by CMS, BC/BS and Alacaid (Alabama Medicaid) for all five levels of new and established outpatients. Now I ask the reader to try to reconcile our average compensation (Table 7-3) with what we get paid per each encounter (Table 7-4) and ask yourself: How may encounters does it take to make this kind of income? Or, how many patients must a physician see, at these rates, to be able to make a decent living? The truth is that another consequence of price control is that it forces physicians to crank up the volume of encounters in order to be able to make ends meet. At present, this is becoming increasing difficult for practices that are highly dependent on CMS, and has led to increasing number of physicians either abandoning medicine, or restricting their practice to non-CMS patients.

Another aspect of medicine that receives little attention during general discussions is the amount of uncompensated work done by physicians. It begins with all the phone calls every physician is asked to answer or to make in regards to patient care. There is the patient who forgot information during his visit and now wants us to stay on the phone with him to discuss matters that may require us to change prescriptions, or order additional tests. Or the patient who got to the pharmacy after being in our office, and there he was advised (see Chapter 10) about the medication we prescribed and wants to renegotiate by phone. Recently, an agent of the Internal Revenue Service (IRS) expressed curiosity about how much we got paid for being "on call" for the hospital. The answer? Nothing! We have to place our lives on hold several times per week and we do not get compensated for the inconvenience. Can we negotiate our terms, or can't we? The truth is that medicine by phone is not only uncompensated work, but also low quality work. However, it is convenient for a subset of the patient population with an entitlement mentality, who insists on the phone being the vehicle of communicating with physicians, without any need for payment for such services. I often wonder what would happened if, in order to speak with the physician, you were automatically charged let's say $9.95 per minute by using your credit card (just like phone sex!). I suspect the number of nuisance phone calls we all get would decrease. I also think that patients would begin to bring their questions written to the office encounters and would pay closer attention to the instructions being given in the office; anything to avoid having to call back and be charged for the conversation!

Finally, let's explore the topic of physician compensation from the point of view of the quality of care delivered. The moment we recognize that physician compensation is identical for all practitioners and based on rigid reimbursement formulas created by the government, rather than by the free exchange generated by a supply and demand system, we obligatorily must conclude that the system views and treats medicine as a *commodity*. This is a critical point to discuss, because of the implications and consequences that it engenders; let me explain further. In economics, a *commodity* is a good for which there is demand and which is supplied *without qualitative differentiation* across the market. In other words, all suppliers of such good are considered to provide the same quality of goods, and therefore are paid equally. This last attribute, known as *fungibility,* is perfectly exemplified in commodities such as wheat, petroleum or copper. Since it is impossible by looking at any of these to know who produced it, their price is identical across the entire market. Accordingly, by paying every physician uniformly, the system has effectively *commoditized* medicine and in the process, it has sacrificed quality. How about another anecdote to illustrate the magnitude of the problem? About seven years ago we opened our own imaging center, a very important endeavor since so much of the practice of neurology depends upon Magnetic Resonance Imaging (MRI) of the brain and spinal chord. At the time, I faced the decision of whether to buy the most sophisticated 3.0 Tesla MRI available to provide the best clinical diagnostic services possible, or to simply be content with the more widely available 1.5 Tesla, with lesser quality images but costing only half the price of the other. I finally decided on the former (my desire to provide the best medical imaging service possible prevailed) despite the fact that I knew this decision would definitely put a financial strain on our cash flow. Why? Because all MRI studies are paid at the same rate despite the quality of the instrumentation, or the quality of the images produced. Thus, here we were generating the same income that we would have generated with the lesser quality magnet, but our instrumentation lease payments were twice as much. Do you find this difficult to believe? I wish I had had a recorder the day we met with the Blue Cross/Blue Shield (BC/BS) representative to discuss our reimbursement rates. Her response to my statement describing the image quality superiority of 3.0 Tesla magnets was: *"We are concerned with payment for services, not with quality..."* She was right! In Alabama, the BC/BS reimbursement for MRI studies is the same whether performed in our center, or in centers with 0.5 Tesla magnets, which provide images of 1/6th the quality of ours, so long as they have filled the proper paperwork of course.

The most important consequence of the commoditization of medicine is that it is a recipe for mediocrity. In other words, why would anyone strive to provide the best medical service possible if the compensation is not commensurate? On the contrary, faced with the prospect of being paid a fixed and discounted fee for services rendered, many physicians succumb to the temptation of making the absolute minimum effort that assures payment. We see this every day, as physicians operating on "survival mode" are slowly replacing the passion for excellence in medicine. By doing the absolute minimum to be able to make a living, physicians have shifted away from their innate creativity, intellectual curiosity, and courage to go against the grain. The physician of the future, product of our current system, is bound to be a public servant who follows the regulatory guidelines for each step of clinical care. Personally, I find this whole idea alarming!

In summary, physician compensation in our country is commoditized, creating little motivation for excellence in care. It is not competitive across markets within our society, creating little incentive for entrance as a practitioner. It is based on a centralized, government-led, convoluted, bureaucratic and inefficient system of reimbursement, which substantially adds to the indirect cost of care and, therefore, the overall healthcare cost. It rewards mediocrity and delays the business cycle of the clinical encounter. Because of all these reasons, any future plan to repair our healthcare system, in order to be successful needs to include an optimization of the physician compensation structure and mechanism; one based on free market ideas and capable of rewarding excellence, so its downgrading effects are reversed.

8

Regulation of Conflicts of Interest

"The irrationality of a thing is no argument against its existence, rather a condition of it!"

Friedrich Nietzsche
German Philosopher, Poet and Composer
(1844 - 1900)

The name Pete Stark (D–California) was largely foreign to me until the late-1990s. However, in the context of the practice of neuroimaging [i.e. the use of a variety of medical imaging techniques such as ultrasound, computed tomography (CT), or magnetic resonance imaging (MRI) for the appropriate diagnosis of neurology conditions], I became acquainted with his name in the context of this U.S. Congressman's introduction of an initial bill that eventually led to three different legal provisions that together are known as the *Stark Law.* These statutes, contained within the Omnibus Budget Reconciliation Acts (OBRA) of 1989 and 1993, as well as the Balanced Budget Act (BBA) of 1995, have been primarily concerned with regulating the extent to which physicians make referrals to entities in which themselves (or direct family members) have a financial interest (i.e. the so-called *"self-referral"*). In principle, the objective of the Stark Law has been to limit the "overutilization" of ancillary services rendered to Medicare patients by curbing financial incentives to "self-referral". Inferentially, the Stark Law subscribes to the assumption that physicians who own facilities in which certain ancillary services [the so-called "Designated Health Services" (DHS)] are delivered, are more likely to inappropriately overutilize them (i.e. order DHS irrespective of whether the patients actually need them or not). As such, the entire regulation has been based on what has been perceived to be a physician's overt conflicts of interest.

The reason I think it is important that we discuss the motivation, conceptual foundation, execution and implications of the Stark Law is that it is a perfect example of how a perceived conflict of interest, in the hands of government agencies and their cronies can easily become the source of an economic stranglehold on a sector of the healthcare system, downgrading it amidst self-congratulatory cheers from the bureaucratic stands. Moreover, it will allow me to introduce the reader to the methodological flaws behind the development of many government regulations, the majority of which do not improve patient care despite the sophistry that leads to their implementation. To this end, in the following pages I will examine in detail the fundamental concept of conflicts of interest, and I will follow this with a step-by-step look at how the Stark Law came to be, paying particular attention to the differences between the rhetoric and the reality that concern this legislation. I will also discuss the political agendas that can be identified behind its various aspects and components. Finally, I will introduce the reader to additional examples of how physicians' actions are preemptively judged by the government in what I consider a most unconstitutional display of *presumption of guilt*.

Personally, I favor the following working definition of a conflict of interest: *"A situation in which an individual involved in multiple interests runs the risk that one of them potentially corrupts another"*. Notice that the definition reads "potentially" rather than a more deterministic adverb like "undoubtedly", "unquestionably", or "predictably". Therefore, it is important to recognize and understand that all conflicts of interest are only "perceived" unless there is evidence that it is consistently and persistently associated with impropriety. This last condition, in my opinion, is a *sine qua non* for the existence of a conflict of interest and precludes the inclusion of occasional, casual or accidental occurrences within the definition. Consequently, a conflict of interest is only operationally present when one can identify a *pattern of behavior* that can be plotted with historical evidence and that displays future predictability. In addition, the nature of the *alleged impropriety* resulting from the conflict of interest must pass critical analysis and scrutiny; the relationship between the two should not have alternative logical explanations that fulfill productivity or excellence models that could also justify the pattern observed. As we will see in the following pages, the latter is a very important point when we consider how expertise in a medical field shapes the choices made by the individuals in that field. Thus, I submit that it is *expected* for certain physicians to order certain tests or medications more frequently than their peers by virtue of their knowledge and experience. I will come back to this point repeatedly as our discussion unfolds in the context of the regulations that presently plague us.

The first stop in our regulatory tour is Stark I, the initial installment of the provisions championed by the good congressman. This was included in the OBRA 1989 and became effective in January 1992.[6] Its introduction resulted from a congressional concern about the implications of physicians "self-referral" arrangements. The end result was that it effectively prohibited physicians from making referrals of Medicare patients for clinical laboratory services to facilities in which the physicians in question (or any family member) had ownership, investment or a compensation arrangement. It also prohibited these facilities from billing Medicare for these services. The details of the forbidden relationships were specifically and precisely defined in the legislative language. Conversely however, the motivation, background, methodology, results and recommendations that led to Stark I left a lot to be desired. Let's look at these more closely. In 1988, Congress mandated the Office of the Inspector General (OIG), Department of Health and Human Services (DHHS), to conduct a study on physician ownership and compensation from entities to which they make referrals. The OIG report, readily available, curiously lists as the background and rationale for their study the following material: a) One editorial in a medical journal, b) Several articles in non-medical publications (e.g. New York Times, L.A. Times, Christian Science Monitor, Wall Street Journal), and c) Four different studies carried out by different organizations (e.g. Blue Cross/Blue Shield of Michigan). Seriously? On one hand, the editorial and the non-medical

---

[6] I warn the reader that following this entire subject becomes confusing when it comes to the dates because, after the various Stark Law phases were passed, they were discussed for several years and the actual federal regulations applicable to Medicare took additional time

articles are simply opinion pieces. On the other, a review of the four itemized studies shows that, at best, they provide dubious results. In any case, the OIG began its project with the notion that facilities with physician ownership or interest have approximately 20-40% more patient referrals than those without. Armed with this information, the OIG studied the topic by means of two physician surveys and by reviewing Medicare B claims annual data for 1987. They also interviewed and consulted state officials, industry representatives, and healthcare "experts". The findings can be divided into three main categories:

1) Physician Interests. Approximately 12% of physicians owned (or had interests) and 8% have compensation arrangements with facilities to which they refer. Physicians invest in a variety of business ventures.

2) Facilities Interests. Nationally 25% of laboratories, 27% of physiology laboratories, and 8% of durable medical equipment (DME) companies have physician interests. Approximately 17% of facilities have compensation arrangements with physicians. The arrangements vary widely by state.

3) Impact on Patient Care. Patients of physicians with interest in facilities get 35-45% more laboratory testing and 17% more physiologic testing than the rest of the Medicare population. This was estimated to cost approximately $28 Million in 1987. There were no differences in the use of DME services due to physician interests.

Can you spot the flaws in the entire exercise? The most blatantly obvious is the fact that the study did not address the issue of quality at all. Before anyone can justifiably scream "conflict of interest" and "impropriety" based on these data, shouldn't they have also examining alternative explanations? For example, in addition to the financial incentives (I have no desire to dispute the fact that physicians have interest in profits just like anyone else), perhaps physicians own laboratory facilities because they have a better understanding of the services offered by virtue of knowledge and experience; perhaps these same two characteristics influence them to own facilities in order to assure that the quality of the services offered is commensurate with what they want for their patients. None of these issues were ever raised in any of the studies, and their relevance has simply been ignored. Another interesting tidbit about the OIG report (and the previous studies for that matter) is the fact that, for every metric, the results uniformly represented a minority of the total practice. Irrespectively of this fact, and at the risk of changing the entire national practice based on that of a minority of players, the recommendations of the OIG were as follow:

1) Medicare:
   a) Require facilities to disclose physician ownership or investment.
   b) Require claims submitted by all entities to contain the referring physician's name and provider number.

2) Policymakers:
   a) Implement a focused post-payment utilization review by carriers.

b) Require physicians to disclose financial interests to patients as a condition for participation.
c) Improve the enforcement of current anti-kickback authorities.
d) Institute a private right of action for anti-kickback cases.
e) Prohibit physicians from referring to facilities in which they have financial interests.

In looking at these recommendations, even I think some are reasonable; for example I have no quarrel with physicians providing full disclosure of financial interest in facilities. However, the one OIG recommendation that became the focus of government intervention was (e). And so, *Stark I was born!* Let me reiterate the irrationality of passing a law: a) Based on a minority of practice, and b) With incomplete assessment of other metrics that may have altered the results (particularly quality). It not only creates an artificial environment by force, but it also sets a precedent for additional government intervention following a paradigm of presumption of guilt. I call to your attention the fact that the OIG never provided any data that would even suggest that the alleged "excess" of referrals was *inappropriate!*

Fast forward just a few years, to the OBRA 1993, in which Stark II made its debut. The basis of this installment of the Stark Law was the so-called Florida study; carried out by the Florida State University under a government contract, it examined how different DHS were ordered in relation to financial arrangements between physicians and the entities that provided them. The authors concluded that there were no negative effects of these financial arrangements with respect to the utilization of hospitals or nursing homes; or for treating rural or underserved populations.[7] They had no definite conclusions about utilization of home health services, DME companies, radiation centers and ambulatory care centers. The trust of Stark II, however, was based on the finding that the patients of physicians with financial interests in independent laboratories, imaging centers and physical therapy centers had higher referral rates. As it pertains to neuroimaging, a subject very close to my heart, the *coup de grâce* came from a 1993 report by the Government Accounting Office (GAO) to Congress, in which they noted that physicians who owned imaging facilities referred larger amount of patients than non-owners; 54% more MRIs, 28% more CTs and 25% more ultrasounds. And so, Stark II extended the "self-referral" ban to an additional list of services (particularly imaging) with the addition of certain provisions, and extended the entire regulation to Medicaid.

Interestingly, Stark II (all three phases) floundered between 1995 when it was included in the BBA, through a presidential veto, and 2007 when it finally became effective. There are some Phase IV regulations that are still being discussed, and the Affordable Care Act (ACA) (i.e. Obamacare) already includes additional provisions that will make the situation even worse. Throughout all of its history, the Stark Law has been nothing more than an assault on the industriousness of physicians, as well as their right to benefit from their clinical and ancillary expertise. As I noted earlier, the law has been largely based on a minority of overall practice, with incomplete assessments that forego the quality

---

[7] Interestingly, despite these particular findings, the Stark Law forbids physician ownership of hospitals outside some very restrictive "safe harbor" exceptions

metric, and the unconstitutional undertone of the presumption of guilt. Under the pretext of "cost containment", the government has unleashed a regulatory maze that is unnecessarily convoluted, wrongfully prioritized, and incapable of adding value to the system.

In this context, I must take a moment to introduce the model of how quality and cost relate to value (Figure 8-1). Although I will expand this further in Chapter 14, the only way to properly address the unfairness of the current

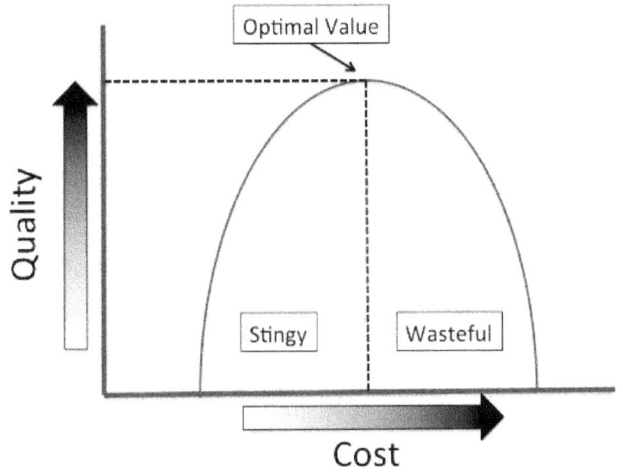

Figure 8-1
Relationship Between Cost, Quality and Value

government approach to this aspect of physicians practice, is to argue my contention that, *without delivering quality services, cost reduction represents a road to mediocrity*. Let's look at Figure 8-1 and the fundamental concept it illustrates. Theoretically, every service (medical or not) can be delivered with excellence and with the highest quality. In turn, such delivery has one and only one precise cost; one at which the delivery of the best quality results in the *"optimal value"* (i.e. the biggest bang for your buck!). Any artificial variation in cost will be accompanied by a reduction of the service quality, either because of insufficiency (i.e. stinginess with inadequate service) or wastefulness (i.e. excessive and unnecessary spending). It follows that simply looking at the cost of anything, without considering its quality, does not allow a proper assessment of the value of the service. And yet, this is exactly what the government and its cronies have done for years! They have considered medical services expenditures and utilization, without factoring their quality (effectively treating them as a commodity as I discussed in Chapter 7), and have concluded that the physicians who have ownership in DHS facilities have led the system to be "wasteful" when in fact, one could argue that the physicians who are not owners of DHS facilities practice *"medical stinginess"* and have shortchanged patients from services they were justified to have.

Perhaps more importantly is the presumption of impropriety that is always embedded into the government analyses. For example, as a neuroimager, I order substantially more MRIs and CTs than the average neurologist and I resent the implications that such a practice makes me a crook! I submit that if you were to examine my career, my education and my experience, you would conclude that neuroimaging is one of my areas of expertise; I have published several books in this discipline, and contributed numerous relevant scientific papers to the neuroimaging literature; I have lectured around the world on this subject, and even served as examiner for neuroimaging certifying organizations. So, should it really be surprising that my practice style is heavily weighted towards the use of neuroimaging? I think not! I also contend that, from my vantage point, it is much more likely that the "typical" neurologist fails to use neuroimaging studies to their full potential. Moreover, mine is not an exceptional example; should we not expect cardiologists to order more electrocardiograms than most other physicians? Or pulmonologists to order more chest radiographs? And, why stop there? Why should physicians be different from *Chefs de Cuisine* who own their own restaurants?

By now, the reader should be wondering why I have chosen to display the term "self-referral" in quotations throughout the chapter. That is easy to answer! Just as with many other government-originated terms, I find it to be yet another federal oxymoron with little logical basis. Descartes must be restless in his grave; *"I self-refer therefore I am?"* Really? *How can we possibly refer our own patients to ourselves?* And, if that is what is meant, where do we draw the line? Should a surgeon who diagnoses a tumor send the patient to another surgeon for an operation in order to avoid the conflict of interest of profiting from said operation? Should surgeons that do not operate, and are not likely to have financial gain from surgery, be the only ones to decide if, when and what type of surgery a patient needs in order to avoid impropriety? Alas, the current state of affairs continues to push the political discourse to empty debates about cost. Likewise, the ACA promises to tighten the grip on this aspect of medical practice, bringing with it additional sanctions and penalties for any deviation from the blueprint of our government-controlled and downgraded system.

Now let's turn our attention to whether the entire Stark Law was needed in the first place. As it turns out, in 1972 Congress had enacted the Federal Anti-kickback Statute (FAS), in order to protect from fraud and abuse of federally funded healthcare related services. This law was further strengthened in 1977 through the Medicare and Medicaid Fraud and Abuse Amendments. The FAS provides criminal penalties for knowingly and willfully soliciting, receiving, offering or paying anything of value in return for the referral of a health care item or service payable under the Medicare or Medicaid programs. Transactions found to be fraudulent are considered felonies punishable by fines up to $25,000 and imprisonment for up to five years. Therefore, amidst our current discussion, it begs the question as to *why would the government embark on creating additional legislation that appears to be redundant to a law that already existed?* This question bothered me from the moment I embarked in writing this chapter. Interestingly, unlike the FAS, which requires proof of intent to induce referrals, the Stark Law was envisioned as a *bright-line prohibition* (i.e. a type of law that does not leave much room for interpretation) of financial relationships between physicians and DHS delivering facilities, without regard to either party's intent or the actual impact on the referral decisions. However, in practice, the Stark Law, in combination with its exceptions, represents a very complex and convoluted set of regulations, far from anything that could be truly considered a bright-line law. At the risk of sounding paranoid, I think the Stark Law has always been about *control*; a politically progressive tool to curb physicians behavior, while limiting their right to a segment of the free market. I submit that it is based on innuendos, veiled accusations of wrongdoing, and the unconstitutional tactic of presumption of guilt, without any solid basis or proof of impropriety.

All that said, despite all of the criticisms I have for the Stark Law, the most egregious example of the presumption of guilt against physicians is the collusion between the Pharmaceutical Research and Manufacturers of America (PhRMA) and the Food and Drug Administration (FDA). Let me set the stage for this facet of my discussion: For as long as

I can remember, I have had a professional relationship with pharmaceutical companies, under a variety of circumstances. As a practitioner I have been visited innumerable times by their representatives, and they have provided me with samples of their product in order for me to give them to my patients as a bridge to their prescription being filled. Also, whenever I have needed answers to an unusual question about their product, one of their professional liaisons has helped me to find the information I needed. As a researcher, I have been both principal and co-investigator of numerous clinical trials of drugs that eventually made it to market. As an educator, I have been sponsored many times by pharmaceutical companies to deliver lectures to various different groups. Yes, I have been to lunch and dinner with industry representatives, and on occasion I have even used one of those plastic pens that carry their logo. Throughout all of these interactions, I have always maintained my integrity and there is no one who can say that they have bought my opinion, or my prescribing practices. I choose the drugs that I prescribe based on the potential benefit they can do for my patients, rather than on how short the miniskirt of the attractive drug representative is. Apparently, however, integrity and track record are not sufficient. Just like every other physician in our country, I am now subject to a "Code of Interactions with Healthcare Professionals" completely based on the presumption that receiving plastic pens or lunches from drug representatives leads to a corruption that translates into inappropriately prescribing practices. Frankly, I must admit that it never occurred to me how rewarding it could be to sell my opinion for a plastic pen or a sandwich!

At this point, you may be inclined to think that I'm making too much of an issue of this subject. Moreover, you may be wondering why I named the FDA as one of the architects of this unfair situation. Let me illustrate how paradoxical some of the changes imposed on us relative to this topic are in regards to the ethics involved. It used to be that, every time I lectured on behalf of a pharmaceutical company, I was able to have the freedom to use any slide and information piece that I wanted. I was free to express my opinion, regardless of whether it was suitable to the company funding the educational program or not. In my mind, this assured that the information I was conveying was personal and that I was not just a mouthpiece for the pharmaceutical industry. The current state of affairs is quite different. In order to lecture on behalf of a pharmaceutical company, outside of programs that lead to continuing medical education (CME) credits and which are regulated differently, any prospective speaker must sign a contract and undergo a predetermined training program geared at assuring that the material being taught is exactly what the FDA determines. Imagine that! After all these years of educating at all levels of the medical profession, we are asked to submit to an indoctrination program and we are handed the information we must convey, actually being told not to share from our personal experience. You might as well record information and hand it to the audience in DVDs that they can watch at their leisure. Needless to say, once these regulations became effective, some of us largely ceased to participate in such a government-controlled (i.e. FDA) and PhRMA-enforced type of "educational" activities. Again, this type of arrangement makes the speaker into a mouthpiece for both entities, and contributes to the brainwashing of the audience by means of choosing information that is politically correct rather than medically correct.

I do not deny that "real" conflicts of interest exist. I also do not deny that fraud, abuse, and dishonesty can be part of the interactions between physicians and the government, or between physicians and the pharmaceutical industry. Frankly, when it comes to physicians found guilty of any of these charges, I say revoke their licenses and throw them all out! My concern is with the generalization made on the basis of individual cases, and with the presumption of guilt with respect to the rest of us who have a clear conscience in both respects. I also have a serious problem with the implication that the honoraria paid to physicians by industry are *in and of themselves evidence* of wrongdoing. Currently, there are private organizations (e.g. www.ProPublica.org) and members of Congress [e.g. Charles E. Grassley (R-IA)] that maintain ongoing investigations into this subject. However, the tone of their findings and the veiled accusations contained within their communications are disturbing and unfair.

In summary, conflicts of interest are potentially unethical situations that may or may not result in impropriety. Despite this caveat, the government has chosen to focus on the convenient concept of cost containment in order to curtail and restrict physicians from engaging in business ventures related to the delivery of DHS to Medicare and Medicaid patients. Such an overreach is based on flawed assessments of a perceived problem, combined with what is a blatant presumption of guilt that tramples the constitutional rights of physicians. These government regulations have also set the tone for similar regulations to take place in the private sector, affecting the relationships between physicians and manufacturers of medications and medical devices. The resulting climate is one that defies any possibility of a free market approach to the delivery of these services, ultimately having a negative impact on the quality and pricing of services. Finally, although I wholeheartedly favor transparency and full disclosure on the part of physicians, I have serious concerns about witch-hunts and unfair punitive behavior on the part of the government and its cronies.

9

Medical Malpractice

"Yep son, we have met the enemy, and he is us"

Walt C. Kelly (as Pogo Possum)
American Animator and Cartoonist
(1913 - 1973)

Malpractice insurance exists because malpractice exists! Make no mistake; we see it every day; we witness it in countless clinical scenarios; we often wonder how is it possible that certain physicians get away with it consistently and persistently. So, in the face of this admission, how do we address the statements made by different groups, some which we otherwise support, that call for *"tort reform"* as one of the most important necessities of any meaningful "healthcare reform"? Well, I submit that, just like anything else in life, there are always two sides that must be considered. In the following pages, I hope to reconcile both sides of the malpractice debate and show that in fact, in order to have a fair outcome, this topic will have to be considered both from the perspective of the physicians as well as from the perspective of the patients. Sounds familiar?

Far be it for me to say that my last statement brings to mind the concept I have been hammering since the beginning of this book: The need to return our focus of medical care to the intrinsic relationship between the physician and the patient (Figure 1–1).

I would like to start our discussion by clearly defining the various components of this subject so we can establish a common frame of reference from which we can further analyze, both historically and prospectively, all the aspects of any relevance. Let's begin with a working definition of medical malpractice: *"A form of professional negligence by act or omission in which a physician provides diagnostic or therapeutic services below the standard of practice by the medical community, incurring in a breach of the duty of care that directly results in harm to the patient, or his death."* Although incidents of medical malpractice may involve *medical errors*, the two terms are not interchangeable. In turn, *tort* is the term applied in common law to any situation in which a person's behavior has unfairly resulted in someone else's harm, suffering, or loss. Although not necessarily and illegal act, a tort affords anyone who has suffered such harm a mechanism by which to recover his loss. In this context, *duty of care* is a legal obligation demanded from an individual (e.g. physician) to adhere to a standard of care that is reasonable and commensurate with that of the community at large. This *standard of care* implies the expectation of an acceptable degree of prudence and caution when discharging the duty of care. In further considering the subject of negligence, the breach of duty in question must be proved to be the *proximate cause* of the alleged injury. Finally, for a malpractice claim to be successful, in addition to demonstrating a *breach of the duty of care* that in fact was the *proximate cause* of an *injury*, it is also necessary that it substantiate the existence of *damages* (monetary or emotional losses). Although in principle the outcome of any medical malpractice claim can be a judgment either in favor or against the physician, a third alternative exists in which the case is *settled* by means of an *indemnity payment* that is conceptually equivalent to payments made based on adverse judgments.

So, what is the current situation of medical malpractice in our country? The most recent data available show that approximately 7.6% of physicians in all specialties have claims made against them every year. However, some specialties are more prone to this experience than others. For example, neurosurgeons average 19.1% and cardiovascular surgeons average 18.9% per year. Conversely, psychiatrists have the lowest rate of claims per year (2.6%) and my specialty (Neurology) ranks close to the mean at 7.5% per year. However, these figures do not tell the entire story, for it is only a small percentage of the claims (mean = 1.6%) that result in indemnity payments. Moreover, there does not seem to be a correlation between the percentage of physicians in any specialty that face a malpractice claim and the proportion of these that end up making indemnity payments. For example, gynecologists have the 12th highest annual rate of malpractice claims but the highest rate of payments (38%). In addition, the data regarding the size of the indemnity payments show that these do not correlate with the frequency with which claims are made. In this respect, pediatricians are at the top of the list, averaging payments in excess of $500,000, but followed closely by pathologists, obstetricians, and neurosurgeons (all three averaging $300,000 to 400,000). Further analysis of the information available demonstrates that, throughout their career, 70-99% of physicians will face at least one malpractice claim, and 19-71% will make at least one indemnity payment. The variability of these figures reflects their dependence on the inherent risks of the different specialties. And so, the evidence demonstrates that only a minority of physicians face malpractice claims on a yearly basis, and that even a smaller proportion of these result in indemnity payments. Still, these results do not consider the indirect cost of litigation, including stress, spent time, added work, and impact on professional reputation. And then there is the National Practitioner Data Bank (NPDB)...

The NPDB was established by Congress as part of the Healthcare Quality Improvement Act of 1986. It is an electronic repository of all payments made on behalf of physicians in connection with medical liability settlements or judgments, as well as adverse peer review actions against licenses, clinical privileges, and professional society memberships of physicians. By law, the NPDB is required to make the information available to hospitals, state licensure boards, some professional societies, as well as to other healthcare entities on their specific circumstances. More recently, in 2010, the Department of Health and Human Services (DHHS) issued a final ruling regarding Section 1921, by which the Social Security Act authorized the NPBD to collect information about negative sanctions imposed by state licensing boards, peer review organizations, and private accreditation bodies against physicians. The importance of the NPBD cannot be overemphasized and has certainly been a matter of concern for the average practicing physician. As we will see in the paragraphs that follow, the argument that physicians in the United States are prone to practice "defensive medicine" in an attempt to avoid malpractice claims and the resulting reporting to the NPBD are at the center of the debate regarding the need for medical malpractice law reform.

However, before we embark on a discussion regarding the merits and fallacies of tort reform, let's go back for a moment and examine the differences between medical negligence and medical error. The context of this comparison is the subject of *frivolous lawsuits*; that is, claims without merit because errors or injuries cannot be verified. It is currently estimated that approximately one third of malpractice claims are not associated with medical errors. Fortunately, the majority of them (about 72%) do not lead to an indemnity payment. In addition, it is only a minority of malpractice claims (less than 5%) that carry no verifiable medical injury. Therefore, if we were to consider the subject of frivolous lawsuits, the truth is that these are too infrequent to have any significant impact. Especially since the majority of them do not ever lead to financial compensation. This is an important point for it has been advanced as a potential component of any serious attempt at tort reform.

So, how do physicians typically respond to the issue of medical malpractice? In one word, *poorly*! There is the natural concern for having to face a malpractice claim, with all its consequences. This is widely regarded as the justification for the practice of *defensive medicine*, also with its consequences. A working definition of defensive medicine is *"an alteration of physician's behavior, diagnostic or therapeutic, motivated by a desire to minimize exposure to malpractice claims"*. Generally, it has been described as taking one of two forms: a) Assurance behavior and b) Avoidance behavior. The former involves actively engaging in practices that are "not indicated" (e.g. ordering tests, prescribing medications, referring for consultations), while the latter relates more to physicians sidestepping the performance of risky procedures or even caring for high-risk patients. It is also possible to find in the existing literature allegations that the undertaking of procedures that are "not indicated" is not necessarily due to physicians concerns with the risk of litigation, but a deliberate attempt at increasing services to create revenue; an accusation that dovetails with our discussion of conflicts of interest in the previous chapter. Regardless of whether defensive medicine results from a litigious or a financial motivation, its prevalence is estimated to be very high, with some studies quoting rates that approximate 80-90%, and resulting in a significant expenditure within the system itself. I would call your attention to the fact that I have qualified the allegedly excessive ordering of tests and procedures within the scope of defensive medicine by referring to these as "not indicated". My reason is simple: It is often difficult for any physician to retrospectively conclude that a test or a procedure was "not indicated", without having been present at the moment the decision was made in concert with the patient.

Now that we have properly set the stage for our discussion, let's consider the important questions we must address regarding medical malpractice. What is the difference between the *apparent* and the *real* occurrence of medical negligence? What role does the current medical tort law play in the downgrading of our healthcare system? Does the current climate justify the practice of *defensive medicine*? What changes could be made so the rights of both physicians and patients are protected, and medical tort law serves a constructive purpose? In answering these questions, I want to bring some balanced perspective to the subject; compare how things are with how they could be; explore how any attempt at tort reform fits into a potential solution to our dysfunctional system.

In the previous paragraphs we indicated that it is only a minority of physicians that face malpractice claims (i.e. 7.6% annually on the average). This percentage is clearly a lot smaller when we factor the total number of patients as well as the total number of encounters per patient, particularly since each of them represents an opportunity for a medical error. However, these numbers refer more to the *apparent* frequency of medical negligence; the fraction of all incidents that result in claims and are the subject of focused attention. But, how about all the incidents that never led to a claim? What is the *real* frequency of medical negligence? As I indicated at the beginning of the chapter, we see it often enough to conclude that the number of claims underestimates the problem. Furthermore, there is also information to suggest that the public at large also underestimates the extent of medical errors. Interestingly, however, a majority of them also support some form of medical malpractice reform. Still, a more important issue to examine would be the true significance of a larger number of real incidents of negligence.

At present, the most widely quoted data regarding medical errors are those reported and disseminated by the Institute of Medicine (IOM) of the National Academies. Established in 1970, the IOM appointed in 1998 the Committee on the Quality of Health Care in America (CQHCA) in order to identify strategies that could lead to improvement of the quality of healthcare in our country. The CQCHA released two separate reports in 1999 and 2001, the former addressing issues relative to one quality concern: *Patient safety and medical errors!* The importance of this report cannot be overemphasized, for it has set the tone for any discussion about medical errors and their impact on our population. It has also provided the platform from which more regulations and re-engineering of the healthcare system have originated. But, do the IOM findings justify the orgy of "quality measures" currently being shoved down our throats? Stay tuned for Chapter 14 in which I will cover these in more detail. However, for the purpose of our present discussion, I think we should critically examine the data in which the IOM based its recommendations, and which deal primarily with the issue of medical errors and negligence.

The IOM based all its arguments and recommendations on the findings of two categories of studies: a) Those reporting on patients experiencing adverse events, and b) Those reporting patients experiencing medications errors. For the purpose of their report, the following additional working definitions were explicitly introduced:

1) Medical Errors: *The failure of a planned action to be completed as intended or the use of a wrong plan to achieve an aim.*

2) Adverse Events: *An injury caused by medical management rather than the underlying condition of the patient.*

3) Preventable Adverse Events: *An adverse event attributable to medical error.*

4) Negligent Adverse Events: *A subset of preventable adverse events that satisfy legal criteria used in determining negligence.*

The thrust of the IOM report is based on two large studies in which medical records for hospital admissions were reviewed, one in New York and the other one in the states of Utah and Colorado. The first of these two was based on a review of 30,121 medical records that led to the identification of 1,133 (3.7%) adverse events, only 280 (0.9%) of which were deemed to be the result of negligence. Interestingly, however, the authors of this study chose to report the proportions of additional findings as relative percentages of the adverse events rather than comparing them to the total as we did above. This is not a small point for it leads to much larger numbers that lend themselves to misapplication by policymakers. For example, the IOM report boasts *"the proportion of adverse events due to negligence was 27.6%"*, a figure they literally copied from the report and which is supposed to represent the relationship between the 280 negligent adverse events and the 1,133 total adverse events. As it turns out, however, a critical look at the original study uncovers an error of calculation because the actual relative frequency of negligent adverse events, as they described it, is 24.7% (i.e. 280/1133*100). Additional comparisons between the reported data (i.e. those used by the IOM) and the absolute numbers that we will discuss further are provided in Table 9-1.

	New York	**Utah**	**Colorado**
Total Cases Reviewed	30121	15000	15000
Adverse Events (AE)	3.7%	2.9%	2.9%
Negligent AE (NAE)	0.9%	0.9%	0.79%
Death Rate from AE	0.5%	0.19%	
Death Rate from NAE		0.079%	

Table 9-1. Absolute Rates of Adverse Events

The second study widely quoted in the IOM report followed the same methodology to study 15,000 medical records in Utah and Colorado. The results are very comparable (Table 9–1) and the methodological shortcomings are very similar to the New York study. In addition to these two studies, the IOM used as its foundation for its recommendations a variety of other smaller studies conducted at single centers, using much different methodology, and with findings that are simply not comparable. Interestingly, the IOM did not mention data from the Medical Insurance Feasibility Study, which encompassed data from 21,000 medical records and was published in the late 1970's. The results could not have been more akin to those of the two other studies described: A total of 4.6% of "iatrogenic injuries" (i.e. caused by physicians), and only 0.8% rate of injuries that could be considered the result of negligence. The other side of this discussion that we must point out is the magnitude of the disconnection between the numbers of negligent adverse events and the number of malpractice claims made. The IOM did not cover this information, which is readily available: *There are 7-10 incidents of negligence for each claim actually made!*

So, what does this all mean? First of all, the data indicate that the problem of medical negligence is not nearly as bad as the public has been led to believe. In fact, a close look at the absolute rates of negligence indicate that the doomsayer tone of the IOM report, its recommendations, and its *"call to arms"* initiative to modify the entire healthcare system (see Chapter 14) to fix a problem that clearly has been blown out of proportion, are largely unjustified. Along these lines, and the risk of getting ahead of myself, let me place the information we have covered in the perspective of the continuum of quality (Figure 9-1). Perhaps the most widely known metric for the ultimate measure of excellence and quality is *Six Sigma* (σ). This is a management system designed to reduce errors in production by applying the notion of having six standard deviations (i.e. six sigma) between the mean value of any process and the nearest specification point. In doing so, almost no items will fail to meet specifications. As such, any process that achieves six-sigma status is one that has less than 3.4 *defects per million opportunities* (DPMO), or a 0.00034% error rate; five-sigma

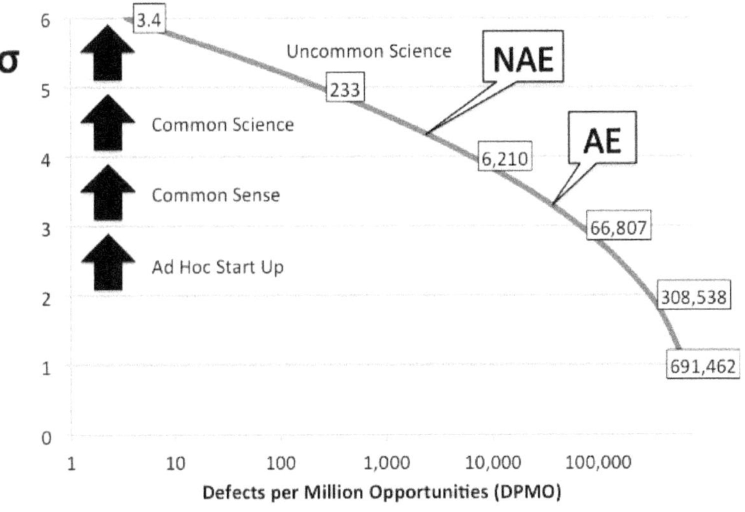

Figure 9-1
Relationship Between Six Sigma and the Quality Continuum

is equivalent to 233 DPMO (0.023%), and so on. Note that, if we plot the historical data we have discussed earlier into our graph, without even having implemented any programs to reduce medical errors, the rate of adverse events approaches four-sigma and negligent adverse events almost score at five-sigma. Moreover, even though I did not plot it in the figure, the death rate from adverse events approaches six-sigma. I submit that these scores are not bad at all as a starting point, a topic I will expand in Chapter 14.

Additionally, our review calls attention to the conceptual difference between the majority of adverse events and the small number of them caused by either medical error or worse yet, by negligence. Let me illustrate this point. As an operator I perform an average of 300-400 interventional procedures per year; the same procedures; the same operator. So, why is it that, in a minority of cases, the outcome is not what I had planned, and the patient experiences an adverse event? The truth is that the presence of an adverse event does not mean that an error has occurred, or that anyone is to blame. Do we make errors? Surely! However, even when errors occur there is no absolute certainty that it will result in an adverse event, and so these terms cannot be used interchangeably.

Another interesting line of though pertinent to the information discussed is how it relates to the practice of defensive medicine. Two plausible points of view can be considered in this regard: a) The rate of negligent adverse events is so low that *it does not justify* defensive medicine, or b) It is so low precisely *because* of it. The former argument, the one I favor, is more of a prospective outlook on the role that such pattern of behavior should or should not have in our professional daily lives. I am inclined to support this argument because I think it is ethically and morally wrong to subject patients to unnecessary tests or treatments, regardless of how "justified" it may seem in the context of the present state of affairs. That said; let me also point out that, although I have never been drawn to the practice of defensive medicine in the strict sense of the word, I consider the prioritization of diagnoses based upon their potential severity (a concept I introduced in Chapter 3) a sound practice, associated with ordering of tests geared at verifying the presence or absence of ominous diagnoses. The price one pays by following this strategy is that frequently the results of these tests are normal (i.e. they disprove the diagnosis of concern). To the uncritical eye, this may lead to the wrongful conclusion that such tests have been "unnecessary" or "not indicated". I contend the opposite: *The result of a test does not in and of itself indicate anything about its reasonableness.* Moreover, from the perspective of the well being of the patient, a *normal study is a good thing!* The second argument, that of defensive medicine being responsible for the low number of negligent adverse events, is simply untenable. None of the information I reviewed could possibly support such notion and, in fact, most of us agree that such practice is wasteful and counterproductive, as it actually exposes patients to unnecessary risks

Does our discussion mean that we should not focus our attention and energy in preventing errors and unnecessary injuries to patients? On the contrary, this should be part of any strategy to provide high quality medical care. My objections with the current initiatives, which I will address further in Chapter 14, are: a) The methodology, and b) The fact that the government is in charge of overseeing the process. I have serious reservations about any project or program designed and monitored by the government. Remember, these are the same people who run the Department of Motor Vehicles (DMV) and the Internal revenue Service (IRS), the former being the epitome of inefficiency, while the latter is the closest organization we have to a totalitarian police body. My discussion above should illustrate how mistaken their assessment of this problem has been. Or has it? Perhaps an alternative explanation is the IOM *purposely* has chosen to report relative rates since their *prima facie* larger values support their alarmist approach to recommendations bound to take us to increasing regulatory control, artificial metrics, and further downgrading of the system (see Chapter 14).

So, what about tort reform? Well, it is imperative that we examine this topic in the context of the conflictive cultural relationship between the malpractice law community and the supporters of patient safety system initiatives. The former is based in the belief that the threat of litigation forces physicians to practice more safely through an adversarial and punitive approach. The latter, on the other hand, involves a softer and "cooperative" type of paradigm. The clash between these two movements impacts many aspects of the problem, including medical error reporting and the acceptance of consequent safety measures. Along these lines, the dissemination by the IOM of their views on medical errors is likely to bring additional litigation by virtue of increasing widespread awareness, and fostering the downgrading of patients' trust in the medical system. One could argue, on the other hand, that since historically only a minority of negligent adverse events result in malpractice claims, such a change may increase the fairness of the entire situation.

In the past, tort reform has been predicated in the context of several categories of proposed changes:

1) Limitation of access to courts. This has included the creation of screening panels designed to discard "frivolous" lawsuits, and shortening statutes of limitation. These strategies are geared at encouraging early settlement.

2) Modification of liability rules. For example, imposing higher standards for breaches of informed consent, or establishing new standards for expert witnesses.

3) Damages reform. In this category, the most popular proposals include caps of damages and limiting attorneys' fees.

4) Alternative mechanisms for solving disputes. These include medical courts, structured mediation and early settlement offers.

5) Alternatives to the negligence standard. Removal of the negligence standard theoretically would morph medical litigation into something similar to worker's compensation.

6) Relocation of legal responsibility. This model would shift the professional responsibility from individuals to organizations (i.e. hospitals).

Every one of these proposed changes has both supporters and detractors. Regardless on which side of the argument you are, it is clear that tort reform must be honestly and fairly considered as part of any initiative to reverse the downgrading momentum of our healthcare system. It is clear that neither an increase nor a decrease of medical claims, in and of itself, will improve patient's safety. Therefore, the challenge will be to find that optimal point where fairness, justice and pragmatism converge.

In summary, medical malpractice exists in our country but at a rate that is anything but alarming. Furthermore, in addressing the problem, one must be careful not to confuse adverse events that do not result from medical errors, from those that do, particularly since the latter are considerably less frequent. There should also be some degree of circumspection when examining the government-driven programs introduced under the banner of "patient safety" since they are largely based on faulty analyses and underhanded use of statistics. Finally, some tort reform must be part of any future solution to our healthcare downgrading problem. However, care must also be exercised to achieve a fair and balanced outcome; one in which injured patients are assured just compensation, consistently negligent practitioners are swiftly excised from the system, and the remaining parties can continue to operate with minimal fear of litigation and no excuse for practicing defensive medicine.

10

Allied Health Professions

"It is better to remain silent at the risk of being thought a fool, than to talk and remove all doubt about it"

Maurice Switzer
American Poet and Writer
(1871 - 1929)

I do not remember any time while growing up at which I either thought or expressed my wish to eventually become a "Healthcare Professional". Still, I am currently by default a member of such an unlikely group. The increased complexity of the medical care required by most patients at the present time necessitates the active participation of a number of individuals with various degrees and who, as a group, are known as *Allied Health Professions*. The original intent of creating specific niches for them within the system was largely that of facilitating the *execution* of a plan of care, conceived, designed, and ordered by a physician. Although many of these professionals continue to play such a function in the daily tribulations of medical care, the last thirty years have seen a progressively expanding role for the allied health professions, regardless of proper justification, and crowding the landscape in such a way that there are instances in which it is difficult to tell who is in charge of what. In the following pages we will discuss relevant aspects of the allied health professions, with particular interest to the differences between the roles they *should be* playing versus the ones they *are* playing. In consideration to the fact that this is a very heterogeneous group, I will try my best to amalgamate some of my comments in search for a cohesive line of thought regarding this topic. The very assortment of educational levels and sophistication needs first to be deconstructed, so we can clearly see the similarities and differences between the various subgroups, providing perspective for our dissertation.

And so, we begin our discussion by providing the reader with a glimpse at the astonishing diversity that characterizes this group. My most recent review led me to identify over 50 different allied health professions, while the Commission on Accreditation of Allied Health Educational Programs (CAAHEP) acknowledges 23 different ones. In looking at these various programs, it is possible to group them into distinct categories. A practical scheme, but my no means an exclusive one, for such grouping is the following:

1) <u>Direct Patient Contact with Formal Degree</u>. (e.g. Pharmacist, Physical Therapist, Occupational Therapist, Speech Pathologist, Respiratory Therapist).

2) <u>Direct Patient Contact without a Degree</u>. (e.g. Phlebotomist, Massage Therapist, Perfusionist, Recreational Therapist, Personal Trainer).

3) No Direct Patient Contact. (e.g. Medical Coder, Healthcare Administrator, Bioengineer).

4) Public Health Related. (e.g. Community Health Worker, Health Inspector, Biostatistician).

As you can see, the group of allied health professions is a hodge-podge of minions that populate the landscape of the healthcare system as part of an ever increasingly convoluted paradigm. Now, this is not to say that they do not serve a purpose or that their presence is not welcome in many instances. My criticism, and the reason why I decided to include this chapter has to do with two important areas in which I think the allied health professions contribute to the downgrading of our system: a) Overreaching into activities that exceed their knowledge or expertise, and b) Openly expressing opinions based upon oversimplified ideas and misconceptions. Both of these problems make the care of the patient more difficult and create significant confusion, which one way or another the physician has to address and resolve. More explicitly, I want the reader to understand that there are a number of allied health professions that have actively pushed for a transformation of their role by overreaching and gaining privileges that are simply in my view not justifiable. Furthermore, even those that stay within the confines of their explicit set of responsibilities, many times interfere (consciously or unconsciously) with the flow of the care of the patient by virtue of volunteering opinions that are well above their "pay grade". This behavior, at best, leads to misunderstandings, although it can result in a schism of the patient–physician relationship. Since it is impossible to address them all, due to their number and variety, I have chosen what I think are the most salient of these infringements to frame our discussion.

Physical Therapy (PT), Occupational Therapy (OT) and Speech Therapy [ST (also known as Speech and Language Pathology)] are, from the perspective of my own specialty, important and necessary for the care of the patients with neurologic disorders. Not one day goes by in which I do not find the need to order one or more of these disciplines to see and look after some of my patients. As a matter of fact, I find their work indispensable in the overall care of any patient with stroke, head injury, and multiple sclerosis, among other neurologic illnesses. Furthermore, as someone who in the past directed an inpatient neurologic rehabilitation unit of 24 beds, in addition to all the acute inpatient work I have done, my contact with these three disciplines has been quite intimate. I strongly believe in the value they bring to patient care but I also have a problem with their own self-image and self-assessment relative to what they bring to the table. The reality is that the nervous system has an incredible capacity for "functional" healing. This may surprise the reader since the commonly held notion is that neurologic injuries do not lead to tissue repair. Although this is largely true, the fact remains that the function lost can be at least partially restored due to the nervous system's ability to compensate or "rewire" itself. I do not want to give the reader the impression that we understand perfectly how this happens because we do not. The different theories advanced, and incompletely studied, that could explain the functional improvement of neurologic patients can be found in the literature under the rubric of *"Neuronal Plasticity"*. While this is most pronounced in children whose brain is not fully developed, the process also occurs in adults. Suffice it to say though, and regardless of the actual mechanism (known or not), following any injury to the nervous system we typically witness functional improvement that varies in degree and latency. Therefore, even though it is frequently impossible to predict how quickly or how much a patient will show return of neurologic function, in the overwhelming majority of cases it is possible to assure them that such improvement *will* occur. Interestingly, such positive change after neurologic injury takes place *despite* what we do and not *because* of it. Surprised? I thought you would be! So, in the context of these revelations, the questions we should be asking ourselves is: *"If the patient is going to improve on his own, what role if any do the three therapy specialties listed have in his rehabilitation?"* and *"How can we justify their involvement in the overall care of the patient?"*

As it turns out, irrespective of what theory we support regarding the underlying actual mechanism, improvement of neurologic function can be greatly *facilitated* by practice. A concert pianist, by practicing many hours a day, facilitates the functioning of neural networks (i.e. specific organized nerve cells connections) patterns that allow him to play symphonies without even thinking how his hands are moving. How? The repeated use of neural networks involved in any type of human activity facilitates their performance. This happens even after neurologic injuries. By now, you should be able to see where I'm heading with this. The neurologically disabled individual benefits from therapy the same way that an athlete benefits from having a coach that points out the best way to carry out activities that facilitate certain neural networks. This is where PT, OT and ST become irreplaceable in the care of our patients. Parenthetically, it is also my opinion that patients who remain partially disabled by virtue of a neurologic injury therefore are in need of therapy intervention without a specific timeframe. This concept is not very popular, and insurance carriers (particularly Medicare and Medicaid) stop funding all therapy efforts after a finite period of time (usually six months) regardless of the results. Unfortunately, this limited coverage mentality is actually supported by some of the statements made by the therapists themselves. And here lies the problem...

Let's begin by discussing the topic of overreaching for additional clinical privileges. One clear example is the fact that, over the last few years, our system has witnessed an insistence of PT practitioners on performing nerve conduction studies (NCS) and electromyograms (EMG); tests designed to assess the anatomic and physiologic integrity of the motor units (i.e. peripheral nerves and muscles), and both traditionally within the scope of neurologic practice. Although I am not a supporter of overregulation or restriction of trade, I must insist that the expertise required to interpret these tests is in my opinion beyond the educational level and qualifications of these individuals. Furthermore, I see absolutely no legitimate indication for these tests to be carried out in order to influence PT practice, except to increase the therapist's income. And yet, the unsuspecting public is exposed to the performance of these tests in what is clearly a substandard form of care.

The problem with OT is slightly different. This is a discipline largely concerned with coaching the patient along the lines of improving his performance of activities of daily living (ADL). These most commonly include grooming, dressing and feeding, among others. Over the course of time, however, the practitioners of OT have extended their scope of work to include making braces that are designed, at least in theory, to reduce contractures (i.e. joint deformities resulting from abnormal muscle tone). The theory, however, is flawed in that it does not consider the fact that the problem is not the joint or, for that matter, the muscles that move that joined. The root cause of abnormal muscle tone lies in imbalances created within the nervous system by injuries that enhance the activity of specific nerve cells. Thus, placing a brace around a specific joint does nothing to change the electrical output of the abnormal (i.e. imbalanced) nerve cells in question. The only way to influence such neurologic dysfunction is through pharmacologic intervention.

Not to be the exception, it is not uncommon to hear ST practitioners discuss with neurologic patients (e.g. those afflicted by stroke or head injury) issues relative to their application of measures pertinent to what they refer to as "cognitive therapy". It is unclear how this came to be but, whatever is meant by "cognitive therapy" is a hoax; it is not based on sound understanding of neurophysiology or neuropsychology. Moreover, it is misleading, confusing and dishonest! Their behavior in the context of this issue demonstrates their limited understanding of how the brain functions. The simple fact that they are involved in the care of someone whose language function is abnormal makes it extremely difficult, nay, nearly impossible sometimes to assess the integrity of cognitive function. The reason for this is because so much of our ability to do so depends on the intactness of speech and language, without which one can never be sure that the patient understands what is being said to him or is able to accurately express what he is thinking.

Beyond the instances of practice overreach that we have mentioned, perhaps a bigger problem is the fact that these individuals do not seem to have sufficient restraint to avoid communicating their opinions with patients and families, irrespective of whether they are accurate or not. It is almost a matter of pride for them to entertain discussions and explanations of issues that do not contribute to the patient's well being or to their overall functional improvement. In Chapter 19 I will introduce my thoughts regarding the topic of patient education, including a critical analysis about the difference between the information they "need to know" versus the one that is gratuitously being shared by a number of minions just so they can hear themselves talk. The impact of conveying an excess of unneeded information cannot be overemphasized, and so I will expand on this and its consequences in due time. Suffice it to say; it is remarkably counterproductive for therapists to engage in oversimplified explanations, many of them filled with inaccurate terminology, that gives them the appearance to be knowledgeable in the eyes of the patient, who simply does not know any better. For example, there are almost weekly occurrences of patients who come to see us for follow-up and mention how their "muscle tone is abnormal" and how the therapist (PT or OT) has explained what needs to be done in order to "bring it back to normal". By now, after completing the last few paragraphs, the reader should be able to identify the fallacy of such a statement. Nevertheless, any incident like that forces us to address it, correct the misinformation, and in the process sometimes give the appearance of being overbearing, arrogant and dismissive. Alas, the alternative is to allow the patient to continue to flounder in a river of misconception.

Another example of an area in which we also run into frequent communication problems relates to the testing of swallowing function in neurologic patients. Again, despite the fact that over the years I have found ST practitioners to be very helpful in this regard, particularly following a stroke or any sudden change in neurologic function, they commonly fail to understand that there is a time and a place for everything. Let me expand on this topic. My experience as a neurologist has shown me (and I would expect it has shown everyone with a similar background) that there are two categorical extremes of patients when it comes to swallowing function; those who can swallow without any difficulties whatsoever, and those in whom the inability to swallow is self evident; unfortunately, the majority of the patients fall somewhere between these two extremes. The ST practitioner's lack of understanding of the evolution and temporal profile of the illnesses in question leads to a mismatch between the required testing and the performed tests. For example, a patient who is incapable of swallowing on Monday may be predictably capable of doing so by Thursday. In this particular case, recommending endoscopic placement of a long-term feeding tube on Tuesday would be premature, and would expose the patient to an unnecessary procedure.

Respiratory Therapy (RT) is another allied health profession of extreme importance in our day-to-day work. This discipline is concerned with the administration of oxygen to patients who need it, the delivery of medications that facilitate breathing function, and the care of mechanical ventilators in intensive care units. Just to emphasize further the close relationship I have had with these individuals, as well as their importance from my point of view, I have thoroughly enjoyed my close collaboration with them both in the intensive care unit and during critical care transport. However, I have found it both surprising and disturbing that, over the last few years, we have seen a slow yet progressive intent on displacing certain responsibilities unto RT. Perhaps the most important example of these being the development of RT-driven protocols for mechanically ventilated patients.

Furthermore, it is also a problem when the RT practitioner discusses with patients and families his idea on what is the best respiratory treatment to be delivered, or what is the meaning of the oxygen saturation (SaO_2) measurements obtained.

Following our previous statements, and despite the fact that it is not considered by some to be one of the allied health professions, I think it is fitting that we take extra time to address issues that are singularly relevant with respect to a prominent professional group: *The pharmacists!* The reasons for such an approach would become clear as our discussion evolves. Before I continue, however, I find it imperative to issue a disclaimer regarding this topic. My youngest sister is a pharmacist; in fact a very accomplished one. In addition, I have many good friends who are pharmacists, whose opinion I respect and with whom I have shared numerous clinically relevant intellectual discussions. That said, I could not in all conscience write a book about the downgrading of the American healthcare system without unmasking a group bound and determined to overextend their reach into the decision-making process of clinical therapeutics. Don't believe me? Just look at around the next time you visit one of the pharmacies of any given national chain and you will see that they now provide "CONSULTATION" (Figure 10-1). It is downright intrusive the way pharmacists wedge themselves between or patients and us, issuing unsolicited and unwanted opinions based on theoretical concepts that do not hold water to the experience of actually treating patients. The motivation for the evolution of pharmacy, from the benign and familiar drug dispensers of the past to the pseudo-clinicians convinced that their knowledge of pharmacology equals their ability to practice clinical medicine, is uncertain. Personally, I favor a combination of egotism and greed, wrapped around by an obsessive identity crisis.

If you think for a moment that I am exaggerating, I invite you to consider the fact that there is a subversive international movement whose sole mission is to promote the expansion of prescribing rights and privileges of pharmacists. In countries such as the United Kingdom, Canada, Australia and New Zealand for example, pharmacists have the legal authority to prescribe drugs. In our country,

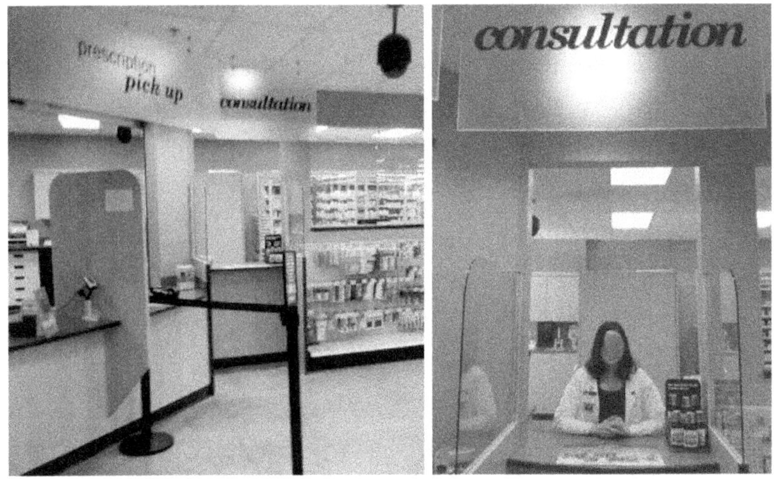

Figure 10-1
"Consultation Window" in a Local Pharmacy

we see an incipient similar movement by virtue of the prescribing rights of pharmacists within the Indian Health Service (HIS) and the Veterans Administration (VA). Moreover, there has been legislation in at least 25 states allowing pharmacists "delegated authority" to prescribed medications under "protocols" sanctioned by the state boards and written by physicians. Although one may think that this is a recent movement, there is evidence of such change in our country that dates back to the 1990's. At present, the champions of expanding the prescribing privileges of pharmacists describe such a movement along the lines of eight different models (Figure 10-2), which vary according to whether they are protocol-based or not, and whether they have a restrictive formulary or not. They are, in order of increasing freedom of practice:

1) Patient Group Direction. This is a written direction signed by a physician and a pharmacist and relating only to the supply and administration of medication to any patients within a defined group.
2) Repeat Prescribing. This involves pharmacists providing medication refills for patients who have exhausted their prescribed drugs prior to their next physician visit.

3) Supplementary Prescribing. In this model, the pharmacist would become the prescriber of medications following a diagnosis made by a physician (i.e. the independent prescriber).

4) Protocol Prescribing. This is the most common form of dependent prescribing and the delegated authority is restricted to a previously agreed protocol.

5) Referral to Pharmacists. Patients may be referred to pharmacists for management of a specific drug therapy by physicians, other pharmacists, or even other patients.

6) Independent Prescribing. The prescribing pharmacist is solely responsible for the patient's assessment, diagnosis and management.

Nonetheless, the most tangible example of the metamorphosis experienced by pharmacists over the last three decades is the role they play within hospitals, particularly academic medical centers, where they have become no less than a Gestapo. At present, it is almost impossible to practice in an intensive care unit (or for that matter even a regular nursing unit) without coming into contact with a pharmacist filled with opinions regarding which drugs should be used in every clinical scenario in order to, most importantly, *decrease the cost of care.* Their authority deriving from committees made up largely by members of the *medical* and *nursing intelligentsia*, these individuals often conduct themselves autocratically, obtrusively, and with blatant disregard of the most fundamental rules of courtesy and professionalism. At this point, the reader may find my remarks rather harsh. However, I invite you to consider how everyday in every hospital in our country, the so-called "Pharmacy and Therapeutics Committees" have meetings in which they decide which drugs must be used largely based on cost containment. Once these decisions are made, with little consideration or input from most of the practicing physicians, the cadre of pharmacists is unleashed unto the nursing units where they proceed to review charts and change orders without ever discussing it with the attending physician of record. In my view, this behavior is underhanded and dangerous, and I am going to use this opportunity to make a case for my opinion.

I want you to envision that, unbeknownst to me, a pharmacist makes a change in one of my patient's existing orders.[8] Then imagine that, in the following hours, a situation

---

[8] This actually occurs daily

presents itself in which there is a change in the clinical condition of the patient (at around, let's say, 3 o'clock in the morning). Such a change would trigger, immediately or shortly thereafter a telephone call to the attending physician, in this case, yours truly. At that time, the information that I would have in my mind to make the next set of decisions includes the medications and treatments I had prescribed myself, before the pharmacist changed them behind my back. Now, without having to hold a degree in Bayesian probability theory or in statistics, most people would agree on the following dictum: *The quality of our decisions is directly proportional to the accuracy of the data in which they are based!* Therefore, in the example above, the probability that I will make a poor decision is relatively high since I will not be basing it on accurate information. The change made by the pharmacist without my knowledge or consent introduces an element of uncertainty that directly jeopardizes the quality of any subsequent decisions. You think this is bad? It is actually much worse! All you have to do is multiply the problem several fold, taking into consideration the concepts we introduced earlier in regards to polypharmacy and the *multi-doctor gambit.* Interestingly, for people who use Evidence Based Medicine (EBM) as a banner to implement changes that benefit them, the fundamental lack of knowledge of the mathematical basis for my argument seems to be a gross deficiency. Furthermore, the legal, ethical and moral implications of these pharmacy-driven changes cannot be overlooked; *should the patient not be made aware that his treatment is being decided not necessarily by his physician of record but by other individuals who may never even have spoken with him?* I would invite the reader to ask the next time he is hospitalized for any reason: Who is deciding what medications are being given to him? Specifically, what pharmacy-driven protocols are being implemented "for his own good"? I encourage the reader to find additional information on this specific topic in Chapters 13, 15, 19 and 21; in combination, all of these will result in a more complete picture of the impact that transforming the scope of pharmacy practice is likely to have in patient care.

In all fairness, it is impossible to conceive that any of these disciplines would have evolved into the condition in which they currently are without acknowledging the complicit role that physicians have had in the entire process. Although this will be covered more extensively in Chapter 13, I find it necessary to bring it into the open so we also begin to take responsibility for the predictable outcome of the abdication of our leadership role within the healthcare system. I contend that it is this sin of omission that has largely translated into many aspects of the system going down a downgrading path of mediocrity. I further submit that undoing and reversing this nonchalant attitude on the part of physicians is a *sine qua non* element for any possible future solution to the problems at hand.

In summary, the allied health professions constitute a heterogeneous group of disciplines that are required in order for medical care to be delivered in all of its current complexity. However, many of them have undergone a progressive transformation highlighted by overreaching of their original clinical privileges with intrusion into areas for which they are simply not qualified. Moreover, they are prone to indiscriminately and uncritically communicate inaccurate and even erroneous information to patients and families, enhancing the confusion that these individuals have in reference to their medical care. Among all of these disciplines, pharmacists appear to be the worst offenders for they in fact almost practice medicine without a license. This behavior is unfair to patients, unfair to physicians, and wholly unprofessional. It is nothing more than another brick in the foundation of a dysfunctional healthcare system. However, we physicians must honestly look in the mirror if we want to find the culprit for such negative metamorphosis of medical care; until we dare do this, we have no right to deny being the root cause of the problem.

HOSPITAL DOWNGRADING

11

The Joint Commission

"A bureaucracy is sure to think that its duty is to augment official power, official business, or official members, rather than to leave free the energies of mankind; it overdoes the quantity of government, as well as impairs its quality. The truth is, that a skilled bureaucracy is, though it boasts of an appearance of science, quite inconsistent with the true principles of the art of business."

Walter Bagehot
English Businessman, Essayist and Journalist
(1826 - 1877)

The Joint Commission on Accreditation of Healthcare Organizations (JCAHO, pronounced *Jay-co*), as this entity used to be known, is more than just a bureaucratic mouthful. It is a "non-for-profit" organization that spawned in 1951 from the merger of the Hospital Standardization Program of the American College of Surgeons (ACS) and similar initiatives by other organizations, most importantly the American Medical Association (AMA), the American Hospital Association (AHA) and the American College of Physicians

(ACP). In 1910 Dr. Ernest Codman proposed a system by which hospitals would track every patient in order to determine whether the treatment they had received had been effective. If not, the hospital would attempt to determine the reason in order to learn the best way to manage similar patients in the future. Three years later, in 1913, the founding of the ACS included Codman's system as one of the stated objectives of this organization. In time, this became known at the College's *Hospital Standardization Program*, and its work helped the introduction of minimum standards for hospitals, the beginning of on-site hospital inspections, and the creation of the first standards manual by 1926.

Following the merger described above, The Joint Commission (TJC, as it is currently known) has progressively become an incredibly powerful organization; one that effectively holds the monopoly (there are some alternative organizations of significantly lesser importance) for the accreditation of a variety of healthcare facilities, including hospitals, home care organizations, nursing homes, behavioral healthcare organizations, ambulatory care facilities, and independent clinical laboratories. At present, TJC accredits approximately 19,000 different healthcare organizations and programs in the United States. In order to earn and maintain this accreditation, every organization must undergo an on-site survey at least every three years (laboratories must be surveyed every two years). A team appointed by TJC and constituted by individuals who either work or have worked within the healthcare system carries out these surveys. In the past, hospitals where notified in advance of the timing of such surveys. However, in response to criticisms, in 2006 TJC began conducting them in an unannounced way. The surveys typically take place sometime between 18-36 months after the previous survey, and they cover the hospital's performance during the entire previous three years. The cost of accreditation for any facility approximates $50,000, plus all expenses for the surveying team members. Along those lines, the reported revenues of TJC are listed in Table 11-1 below:

	2007	2008	2009	2010	2011
Revenue	$148,993,050	$167,203,205	$165,434,965	$169,705,538	$180,459,065
Expenses	$148,073,342	$161,941,438	$152,520,781	$156,200,266	$163,020,697
Ex Revenue	$9.039.954	$6,767,312	$12,914,184	$13,5050,272	17,438,368

Table 11-1. Revenues and Expenses of TJC

Yes, those are hundreds of millions of dollars! In addition, TJC reported additional yearly revenues from investments amounting to about $4.5 Million per year. This information illustrates the "profitability" of TJC. Parenthetically, since the reader may be inclined to ask, *"But, isn't TJC a nonprofit organization?"* I think it is important that we take a moment to discuss this issue, not only because of what it represents for TJC but because it is also relevant to similar organizations that carry out the bidding of governmental healthcare agencies. Technically speaking, TJC is a "nonprofit" organization [i.e. Title 501(c) of the Internal Revenue Tax Code]. However, and perhaps because I think a small dose of paranoia is a healthy thing (and just as Andy Grove's accurately noted in his iconic book *"Only the Paranoid Survive"*), I have a considerable skepticism of these types of organizations. From the financial point of view, all income that a legal entity receives constitutes REVENUE and all outlays of money constitute EXPENSES. Any positive difference between these two constitutes PROFIT. In the case of the non-for-profit organizations, the latter term is substituted for the euphemistic one of EXCESS REVENUE. Again, changing the label does not materially change the fact that there's more money coming in than going out! The real differences are: a) The fact that no taxes are assessed, and b) The fate of the excess revenues. Therefore, although theoretically no one in particular "pockets" the difference between revenue and expenses, there is no reason why the organization cannot distribute these monies in terms of bonuses, or use them for investment. Hence, I want the reader to pay close attention in the future, every time one of the numerous organizations intricately involved in the healthcare system boasts about being a nonprofit entity [i.e. 501(c)], and I encourage a similar measure of skepticism about the altruistic nature of their activities.

The mission of TJC, as it has been stated is *"To continuously improve healthcare for the public, in collaboration with other stakeholders, by evaluating healthcare organizations and inspiring them to excel in providing safe and effective care of the highest quality and value."* Wow! This is the type of statement that appeals to all the noble intentions and pushes buttons within everyone in our community in order to gain widespread support and justify all sorts of activities. Personally, I have grown quite skeptic about this type of initiatives, especially when they are tied to government intervention. Think about it! Even though accreditation by TJC is a voluntary process, it is practically impossible for any healthcare organization to receive payments for services rendered to patients covered by Medicare or Medicaid without having it! And so, TJC accreditation becomes one more stumbling block in our downgraded health care system, simply by creating additional regulations that add operational sluggishness with a questionable beneficial impact on patient care. In Chapter

14, I will expand on the various measures that are forced on the current practice of medicine under the banner of *"Improving the quality of care and the safety of the patients"*. I intend to show that all of these programs are no different than other social interventions the government conducts, endorses, or coerces with the excuse that *"it is looking out for us!"* In the next few pages, however, I would like to take a critical look at TJC and contrast their intended activities with the reality of our current state of affairs.

Let's start by looking at the stated "benefits" derived from accreditation by TJC, as follow:

1) Helps organize and strengthen patient safety efforts. I do not have a major problem with this potential benefit. It seems reasonable that any organization that can assist with organizing efforts according to some methodical paradigm probably provides value added to some degree. However, the statement does not guarantee outcome since it emphasizes a support role for TJC.

2) Strengthens community confidence in the quality and safety of care, treatment and services. This statement is misleading since it does not take into account the self appointed character of TJC, and assumes that the acceptance by the Center for Medicare and Medicaid (CMS) is a *de facto* badge of excellence. However, as we will discuss repeatedly throughout this book, the general assumption that "Government knows best" is completely unfounded and devoid of historical justification.

3) Provides a competitive edge in the marketplace. I found this statement somewhat puzzling because it underscores a conflict of interest. Let's analyze it in the context of the

Vision of TJC: *"All people always experience the safest, highest quality, best-value healthcare across all settings."* So, if the ultimate goal is to improve the quality of care and the practice safety of all organizations, then doing so will result in all of them being equal, canceling any potential "competitive edge" that any one of them may want.

4) Improves risk management and risk reduction. This statement is excessively categorical. Yes, I admit that concentrating efforts in process' improvement may decrease certain risks but I am not convinced that the focus of TJC leads to such an achievement consistently or persistently. Furthermore, as we will see later in the book, there are unintended consequences of a government sanctioned TJC takeover of how medicine is practiced.

5) May reduce liability insurance costs. In my view this is nothing but a sales pitch; One based on the notion that complying with regulatory mandates would be perceived by medical insurance carriers as a sign of increased quality and reduced risk, therefore leading to less expensive premiums. Furthermore, it also suggests that such compliance may become a defense weapon in case a malpractice claim is brought against the organization. Although these assumptions may be true, the outcome cannot be a predictable reduction of liability insurance due to the not so apparent expenditures relative to handling of malpractice claims.

6) Provides education to improve business operations. This is also a very elusive "benefit". There is no doubt in my

mind that decreasing variability is a very worthy operational goal for many businesses. However, the drivers of our operational paths in medical care can be so artificially manipulated by government (and in this case TJC), that efficiency does not necessarily result in the best outcome for the patient. In my experience, the opposite is more commonly true. As we will see in other chapters, the implementation of programs such as those championed by TJC cannot be carried out without the inclusion of numerous activities that add no value, even though they most certainly add work (e.g. forms).

7) Provides professional advice and counsel, enhancing staff education. This is probably the most disingenuous of the so-called "benefits" of accreditation by TJC. I submit that it combines the inadequacy of TJC advisors and counselors, with the bias of the information that is being provided as "education". In other words, TJC provides organizations with the information required to fulfill the needs for the accreditation process, and it does so through individuals who are already indoctrinated into how such information fits into the accreditation process (not the actual care of the patient).

After all of this is said and done, I find it difficult to have a clear picture of how much better any organization is by simply having TJC's *Golden Seal of Approval™*. Alas, it is even less clear how its patients actually benefit from such a feat.

In addition to accrediting organizations, TJC also awards Disease–Specific Care Certification (DSCC) in the treatment of illnesses such as chronic kidney disease, chronic obstructive pulmonary disease (COPD), heart failure, diabetes and stroke. I could undertake another analysis of the "benefits" of TJC certification in any of these illnesses, but the reader is bound to quickly find it redundant, since it follows the same pattern of thinking that led to my conclusions about the accreditation process. Suffice it to say, they constitute an assortment of motivational declarations, sales pitches, wishful thinking, and half-truths about the impact of a regulatory stranglehold on quality improvement. The DSCC provides the framework for the day-to-day quality indicators and measures we will discuss in Chapter 14. Items all that have slowly been pushed into the tapestry of medical care with the pretext that they help improve the quality of outcomes and the safety of the patients.

The governing body of TJC is the Board of Commissioners (BOC), which provides policy leadership and oversight. The BOC meets three times per year, plus a fourth meeting dedicated to strategic planning. It consists of 32 voting members with diverse backgrounds within the healthcare system. The present BOC includes thirteen physicians (i.e. individuals with a medical degree), only four of who practice medicine in the strict sense of the word. The remaining nine include four senior faculty members of medical education institutions, and another five who hold full time administrative positions in various organizations (including the President of TJC). The remaining members of the BOC include dentists, nurses, attorneys, non-medical doctors (i.e. Ph.D.), business officers, and bureaucrats. In general, the BOC composition includes representatives from TJC's corporate members: AMA, AHA, ACS, ACP and American Dental Association (ADA).

Now that we have exposed the claims made by TJC about how beneficial their accreditation and certification processes are to healthcare organizations, and having also explored the diversity of its leadership, it is time to address how TJC focuses its scope of practice. The centerpiece of TJC accreditation process is the surveys. As I noted earlier, these are presently conducted without the organization being forewarned when they will take place. The surveys are primarily designed to assess how the organization complies with TJC performance standards. The latter vary according to the type of organization being surveyed and, out of sheer pragmatism, for the purpose of our discussion I will refer to those pertaining to hospitals. It is said that TJC develops its performance standards in consultation with healthcare experts, providers, measurement experts, government agencies, purchasers and consumers, and they cover key functional areas, such as Emergency Management, Environment of Care, Human Resources, Infection Control and Prevention, Information Management, Leadership, Life Safety, Medical Staff, Medication Management, National Patient Safety Goals (NPSG), Provision of Care, Treatment and Services, Record of Care, Treatment and Services, Rights and Responsibilities of the Individual, and Waived Testing. The development process consists of a fairly bureaucratic method that includes multiple approval steps by diverse advisory groups and internal committees, and final approval by the BOC. Each accredited organization receives a free print copy of the pertinent Standards Manual as well as access to the electronic version (i.e. E-dition). Non-accredited organizations interested in the manuals may purchase them individually.

In addition, as of 2010, TJC categorized its performance measures into *accountability* and *non-accountability* measures. The former are supposed to have the greatest impact on patients' outcomes and, to be considered such, they must meet certain criteria:

1) Research. The presence of strong scientific evidence of their effect on patient outcomes.

2) Proximity. The measure is closely connected to the outcome that is intended to affect.

3) Accuracy. The measure actually measures that the process being assessed is completed.

4) Adverse Effects. The measure minimizes unintended negative consequences.

The non-accountability measures are considered more suitable for secondary uses (e.g. education). Some of the previous non-accountability measures are being slowly retired. In the future, TJC is supposed to only adopt accountability measures for its ORYX® program. The latter was introduced in 1997 as an initiative to integrate outcome and performance measures data into the accreditation process. This set the stage for future collaborative work between TJC and CMS, as we will cover more in depth in Chapter 14. As of January 2012, TJC accreditation will require hospitals to meet a minimum of 85% compliance rate for accountability measures.

The accreditation process begins when an organization submits an application to TJC, thereby providing all type of information relevant to their operations. Following review of the application, TJC schedules an unannounced (with a few exceptions) on-site survey. This is supposed to be tailored to the specific organization, its length limited by the information supplied in the application. The way TJC touts the on-site survey as focusing on "continuous operational improvement in support of safe and high quality care, treatment and services." The agenda of a typical survey includes hospital tours, conferences, meetings, and orientation sessions. Most importantly, the cornerstone of the survey is the application of *Tracer Methodology* to the assessment of patient care. Tracer methodology allows the surveyors to pick actual patients and follow them through the entire hospital experience.

Once the on-site survey is concluded, the surveyors have an exit interview with the organization and share their preliminary findings. Then the information is sent to TJC where one of three decisions is made: Accreditation with Follow Up Survey, Contingent Accreditation, or Preliminary Denial of Accreditation. This recommendation is moved through the organization until TJC Accreditation Committee assigns the final decision on accreditation.

Up to this point the reader must think: *"So, what's the problem?"* It all seems so noble (i.e. quality and safety) and organized! I admit that, at first sight, TJC appears to be the bastion of excellence in healthcare; an unparalleled organization with the best interest of the patients as its primordial driving force. However, when things looks too good to be true... ...they usually are!

The criticisms of TJC abound. Let's start with the conceptual issue of it being a monopoly. Although this is disputed, since there are other organizations that also provide certification of healthcare organizations, most notably the Healthcare Facilities Accreditation Program (HFAP) and Det Norske Veritas (DNV), the truth is that in practice TJC rules! Historically, in 1966, the federal government gave *deeming authority* (i.e. the authority to certify organizations on their behalf) to TJC and this was maintained until 2008, when such a designation was made available only via application. Personally, I think this change was directed by the government in order to protect TJC from being vulnerable to antitrust litigation. Needless to say, however, TJC has continued to have deeming authority through the years. Not surprising, considering the fact that the organization has over $17 Million in “excess revenue” per year. So, even though there are indeed other accrediting organizations, the lion’s share remains with TJC and its long relationship with CMS makes it very influential in many spheres of government related healthcare activities.

In the past, there have also been significant criticisms about the fact that TJC accredits about 99% of the organizations that it surveys. The perception that TJC accommodates its paying customers is not without some merit. I remember how, before 2006, scheduled on-site surveys took place in the various hospitals I have worked through the years. We used to see a barrage of activity designed to make the hospital compliant with the performance standards. Problems we had been complaining about for months to the administration of the hospital would get fixed overnight; the floors would be made shinny; stray wheelchairs or hospital beds would not block emergency exits; laboratory results would be promptly posted in charts; emergency medications would be made available at the bedside in a timely manner, and so on. Frankly, there were times when we asked ourselves if we were in the same hospital we had been one week earlier. If you were really unlucky, you would bump into TJC surveyors as they were being ushered by members of the hospital administration and they would pause to ask some asinine question that required either a bureaucratic or a self-evident answer. They would spend two or three days touring the hospital and, almost immediately afterwards, things would go back to the way they were prior to the survey. Invariably, the hospital in question received accreditation by TJC! This pattern repeated itself in every single hospital I have ever worked, and cemented my view of an incredible hypocritical and collusive process that passed for the model of quality.

After 2006, TJC switched gears, and the on-site surveys are now conducted without any forewarning to the organization being surveyed. You would think that, if my comments were off base, this procedural change would have

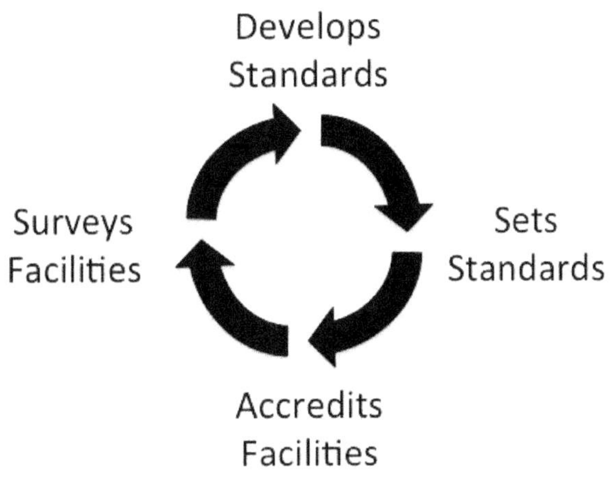

Figure 11-1
TJC Cycle of Control

resulted in a tougher paradigm, with greater potential for failed on-site surveys. Think again! Since this change was instituted, TJC claims that the average number of hospital deficiencies increased from three to seven, and the proportion of hospitals on conditional accreditation jumped from 1% to 2.8% (2007 Information). Really? Are we supposed to be impressed? I think not! Hospitals have continued to be accredited by the dozen, the gears of the process continue to churn, and the hospitals continue to pay their fees to be "accepted" by the government agencies: It is nothing but a rigged card game!

The business model of TJC is exceptional and constitutes a *"cycle of control"* (Figure 11-1). TJC develops the standards, "educates" facilities on the standards, then surveys the facilities and accredits those that "comply" with their standards, all for a nominal fee. Ah! It then develops additional standards that are included in subsequent follow up on-site surveys, and the cycle restarts. It is a conveyor belt of income! Furthermore, its collusive relationship with CMS makes this nothing more than a cycle of government-outsourced control. Make no mistake; this is nothing more than the government using cronies to do its bidding by enforcing dogmatic control.

In summary, TJC is an organization that was created with very lofty goals but, like many other great ideas I have discussed through the book, the final product is nothing but a distortion of the original intent. It is a pseudo monopolistic and "nonprofit" organization, whose finances are consistent with a very profitable scheme; one that hides behind the rhetoric of quality and safety, and operates with impunity by means of bureaucratic and shady tactics. The downgrading effect of TJC on the healthcare system is palpable in every form we are asked to fill in order to comply with regulatory requirements. This is nothing more than another step in the indoctrination and brainwashing we are being subjected as part of our daily activities.

12

Nursing Leadership

"Be a yardstick of quality. Some people are not used to an environment where excellence is expected."

Steve Jobs
American Designer, Businessman and Inventor
(1955 - 2011)

I distinctly remember when I was a resident in neurology how good our head nurse in the Veterans Administration hospital was. The neurology ward encompassed 45 beds, almost always occupied by individuals affected with a variety of neurologic illnesses, both acute and chronic. Any day of the week, there were three neurology residents rotating through that service, assessing patients, requesting diagnostic tests, and writing therapeutic plans. In order to maintain some sense of sanity amidst the potential chaos created by an overwhelming number of clinical issues that constantly popped up, the nursing staff needed to be held to a set of standards based on discipline, expertise, and accountability. The person in charge of these nurses could not have been someone without the experience, skills, and leadership ability to assure that all clinical tasks were completed in a timely and thorough fashion. Our head nurse fulfilled all those characteristics and that made her successful in all counts. It is therefore not surprising that those of us who "grew" within this era and under these circumstances, would take it for granted that, to succeed as the head nurse of *any* hospital nursing unit would require similar standards.

However, we no longer have "head nurses". The current job title for someone who runs a hospital nursing unit has evolved through "nurse manager" to the current fashionable appellative of "nursing unit director", or "nursing director" for short. Just as I have mentioned elsewhere in the book, these changes in title (very likely introduced by the so called *"Human Fulfillment Movement"* I referred to in the Introduction of the book) do not carry with them the same personal attributes described above, or the same job description. Moreover, if anything, they have resulted in downgrading of the quality of the bedside nursing leadership within hospitals. So, while in the past the individuals who were offered the position of "head nurses" arrived at such an offering by having been the best of the best at the bedside, at the present time anyone with the right bureaucratic credentials can make it to "nursing director" without being competent at carrying out the most basic nursing tasks. The reader may think that I am exaggerating but I assure you that were we to ask many a "nursing director" to place an intravenous cannula, or an indwelling bladder catheter (i.e. Foley), it would not be surprising if neither of these two tasks could be carried out proficiently. Thus, what we have today is a situation in which the so-called "nursing leaders" are not necessarily the best of the best in nursing but rather those individuals who have collected a series of degrees that entitle them to be part of an ever expanding bureaucratic machinery whose underpinnings control hospital operations.

I am and have always been of the opinion that the leader of any group should be the individual who acquires such a position on his merit, and relative to his performance in the context of the overall mission of that group. Perhaps it is the way my education took place, or the years I spent in the U.S. Army, but I do not see how it is possible for someone without competence or experience in a certain field to lead others and be able to provide mentorship, supervision, feedback, and education. This ideal leader, exemplified by the concept of the *Akela* of the Boy Scouts (a term borrowed from the name of the leader of the wolf pack in Rudyard Kipling's *The Jungle Books*) and implying a symbol of wisdom, experience, and competence above and beyond the basic standard, would seem to me to be the one everyone aspires to be. Instead, at the present time, we are more likely to find that the "leaders" of nursing are largely out of touch with the reality of the bedside. It is in fact the introduction of such pseudo-leaders that makes it possible for the system and for the *nursing intelligentsia* to influence the daily practice of nursing in such a negative way that it dilutes the meaning of such a noble profession.

The downgrading of the nursing units leaders is palpable in every day practice. It sets the tone for the performance and behavior of all nurses in the unit. Devoid of a true leader, and burdened by regulatory requirements that distract them from their true responsibilities, nurses operate like wound up toys that bump into walls and bounce back... ...just to bump once more against the opposite wall! They have no one to turn to for real mentorship and guidance, and are forced to simply follow predetermined nursing "protocols" lacking the need for judgment and reasoning. In addition, once the leader is unable to properly assess the presence or absence of clinical excellence within the nursing unit subculture, two things happen: the nurses do not strive for such a state of practice, and when they are confronted with difficulty, they pass the buck to someone else (Figure 12-1). Sadly, the system has been padded to protect the nursing leaders so they don't need to come out of their precious committee meetings. How? Well, for example, if the nurse cannot get an intravenous (IV) catheter inserted all she

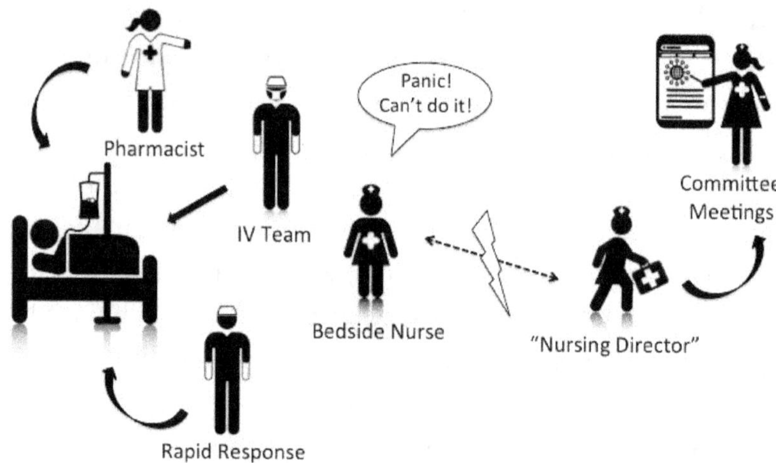

Figure 12-1
The Role of the "Nursing Director"

has to do is call for the "IV Team", whose mere existence guarantees this skill disappears from the scope of bedside nursing practice. Another example of this padding of the system to displace responsibility and avoid uncovering the unit's leadership deficiencies involves summoning Rapid Response Teams any time there is a perception of trouble; a topic I will cover further in Chapter 15. Thus, we are left with a situation characterized by nursing units running amok and simply existing from one 12-hour shift to another.

The problem of the inadequacy of nursing leadership does not end up at the nursing units but expands to those layers of middle management that pervade the numerous committees apparently necessary to operate a hospital. I find it somewhat paradoxical that a profession whose primary goal at its inception was to provide direct care for the suffering, has its so-called leaders so disconnected from actual patient care that they spend their days going from one committee meeting to another, taking part in decisions that have already been made by hospital administrators above their pay grade, or simply juggling unimaginative ideas that they have either read in third class nursing journals, or have heard from peers with their same handicaps. The subculture at these levels is one of cronyism, self-importance and mutual encouragement, almost like a cult in which they compulsorily believe their own rhetoric as if it were gospel. It almost does not matter what the truth is, once a decision has been made by one of these committees, it rapidly becomes integrated into "protocols", and is accompanied by the design and distribution of more forms that the clinical staff is required to complete, all with the absurd excuse that it improves quality. Throughout the book the reader will come across discussions of various topics that involve these middle management nursing "leaders". If it not exactly clear whom I am speaking about, let's go ahead and expand on this concept.

The typical nursing "leader" I am discussing is an individual who has gone to nursing school and has advanced further, having obtained a Masters degree in either nursing or some other discipline. It is likely that this person has spent some time at the bedside, in one or another clinical environment. In my experience, the overwhelming majority of them did so only while getting advanced degrees (their main goal in life) and they were not very good at bedside nursing in the first place. Some claim otherwise, but the truth is readily apparent as soon as they open their mouths. Along the way, they clearly have drank the Kool-Aid® necessary to qualify for all those administrative positions that exist between the Director of Nursing (DON) and the bedside nurses (figure 12-2). That is, they have embraced the touchy feely philosophy that includes patient satisfaction as the ultimate metric for quality and "educating" patients even

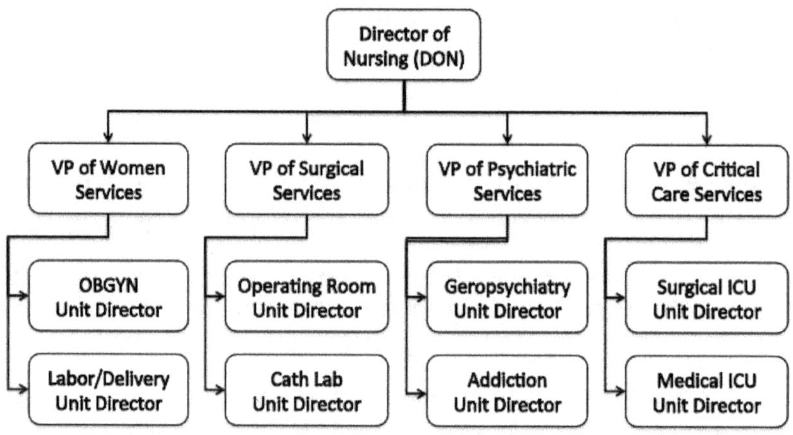

Figure 12-2
Example of Organizational Chart for Hospital Nursing Leadership

when the information provided is inaccurate, incomplete and irrelevant. Just one more box in the list checked! They have utterly important titles such as "Vice-President of Operations" or "Service Line Director" and they earn six figures yearly salaries without exposing themselves to patients' bodily fluids or even the touch of a human being. They have access to an endless supply of continental breakfasts and "working" lunches as part of their committee meeting attendance requirements, and they are phenomenally competent at shuffling papers. They spout out statistics without remorse; numbers they have been forced to memorize since they cannot differentiate between the *mean* and the *median* of a population, or how the Poisson distribution of incoming patients would affect a newly open emergency ward. Oh oh! Maybe I went a bit too far in that last commentary and lost you too. Suffice it to say, their egos *"write checks their bodies can't cash!"*

One of the most laughable aspects of nursing

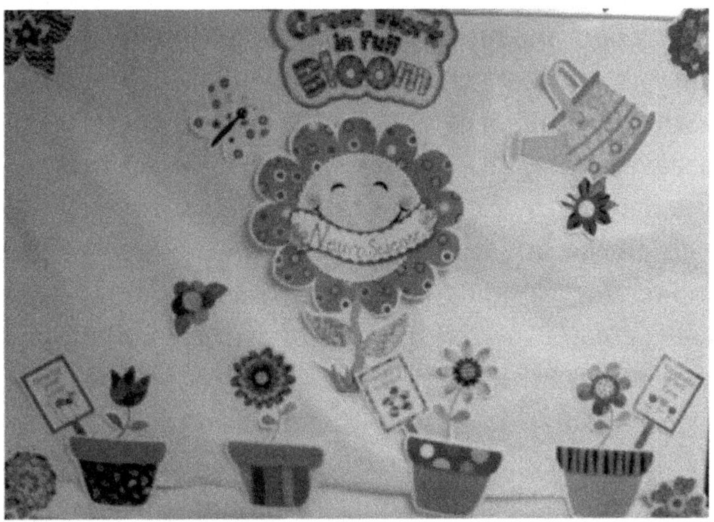

Figure 12-3
Motivational Board on the Hallway of a Nursing Unit

leadership as we presently witness it, is the grammar school approach to their attempts to motivate nurses throughout the hospital (Figure 12-3). As you can see from the picture, this strategy takes the form of rather childish cut-and-paste boards placed ubiquitously throughout the hospital to make nurses feel good about themselves. I am of the opinion that if you treat adults like children, they will oblige you and behave as such. Therefore, it should not be surprising that nurses often lack professionalism and logical prioritization of their responsibilities. This is somewhat paradoxical since, traditionally, the nursing community as a whole has been adamant about being considered "professionals". Meanwhile, they continue to engage on such daily puerile behavior that can hardly be respected by others. Examples of this type of conduct are everywhere and underscore how weak the foundations of nursing leadership truly are.

One particular topic within the nursing leadership culture that we want to cover in our present discussion is that of *case managers*. A product of the introduction of *Managed Care* in the early 1970's, and although technically not in the nursing "chain of command" (Figure 12-2), the overwhelming majority of hospital case managers are nurses who have undergone some type of additional training and now earn up to six figures steering the care of patients though all the bureaucratic hurdles so the hospital can get paid for the patient's treatment. Imagine that; we have actually created an entire line of work, another layer of bureaucracy, to assure all the governmental (and by inference insurance carriers') needs are met, whether they make any clinical sense or not. For example, there is presently an incredibly stupid regulation that requires for the "status" of certain hospitalized patient to be designated (i.e. labeled) as either "INPATIENT", "OUTPATIENT" or "OBSERVATION" in order for the patient's care to be paid (i.e. payment is denied if the wrong "label" is assigned to the patient). Now, this occurs irrespective of the fact that it is *the exact same patient, receiving the exact same service, in the exact same place, by the exact same people, regardless of the label assigned*. Does that make any sense? Does it not strike you that this labeling process is just as beneficial as rearranging the chairs on the deck of the Titanic? Well, guess what? It is the responsibility of case managers to see that the "acceptable" label is entered in the medical record and, to that end, they downright pester the rest of us at all times of the day or night because the physician is required to be the one to designate the status of the patient. Thus, it is not unusual to be called in the middle of the night to fulfill a task we find menial, irrelevant, unimportant, and distracting. Moreover, this topic is persistently and consistently brought up into the priority list of the queries we must endure every day when we make clinical rounds. And our politicians and bureaucrats have the nerve to wonder about the escalating cost of care! So, what does it take to become a case manager? It is possible to enter the world of case management by way of a baccalaureate program in Social Work but I will not dwell on this aspect of the field. Picking up where we left on Chapter 5, a registered nurse (RN) can become a case manager by following one of two paths: a) Certificate Programs in Case Management, or b) Master's Degree Programs in Nursing Case Management. The former spans 6-8 weeks during which the candidate is exposed to instruction on case management in the community and healthcare facilities, life care planning, clinical ethics and legal responsibilities. The latter, evidently more complex, exposes the candidate to a two-year program that encompasses biostatistics, analysis of health policy, financing of healthcare, evaluation and quality assurance methods. So there you have it; another accelerated path to an advanced nursing degree; another ubiquitous "healthcare professional" in the landscape of our downgraded system.

I now want us to turn our attention to *Magnet Hospitals*, one of the biggest scams in nursing leadership. The Magnet Recognition Program (MRP) was created in 1990 by the American Nurse Association (ANA), and has been managed by its subsidiary the American Nurses

Credentialing Center (ANCC). It is considered the highest recognition in nursing excellence and it is awarded to organizations that allegedly provide excellence in nursing. In fact, the ANCC claims *"Magnet Hospitals have higher percentages of satisfied RNs, lower RN turnover and vacancy, improved clinical outcomes and improved patient satisfaction."* Seriously? Why would anyone think that nursing satisfaction is a metric for quality of care? Do we want satisfied nurses, or do we want competent nurses? This summarizes how off the mark this whole project is. Then there is patient satisfaction as a primary metric; another misguided concept that has transformed medical care into a "hospitality industry". I intend to cover this topic at greater length in Chapter 18, so I will not dwell on it too much at this time. Suffice it to say; all we have left is to ask the question: *Does the MRP truly improve the quality of clinical outcomes?*

Let's begin our analysis by looking at the source. The entire MRP concept originated from a study commissioned by the American Academy of Nursing (AAN) in 1981, following the recommendation of a task force it had created in order *"to examine characteristics of systems impeding and/or facilitating professional nursing practice in hospitals"*, and motivated by the serious nursing shortage of the 1970's. That is why the issue of nursing satisfaction is so prominent in the ANCC's statement; it was always about nurses wanting to work in specific places, not about the quality of care; about happiness not competence! The introduction of *"improved quality of clinical outcomes"* came later; most likely because of the need to justify the program's existence once shortages were not as much of a problem, and certainly based on pseudoscientific research. Do you find my comments insensitive? Let's then discuss the particulars of the MRP. Parenthetically, I should mention that I have practiced in a hospital with MRP designation, and in another that is currently pursuing this path.

The MRP is based on the 14 characteristics (i.e. "Forces of Magnetism") the original study found to be of importance in attracting and retaining nurses (i.e. like a magnet!). These Forces of Magnetism (Table 12-1) are organized into five components, as follow:

1. Quality of Nursing Leadership	8. Consultation & Resources
2. Organizational Structure	9. Autonomy
3. Management Style	10. Community & Healthcare Organization
4. Personnel Policies & Programs	11. Nurses as Teachers
5. Professional Models of Care	12. Image of Nursing
6. Quality of Care	13. Interdisciplinary Relationships
7. Quality Improvement	14. Professional Development

Table 12-1. Forces of Magnetism

1) Transformational Leadership. The idea here, as stated by the ANCC is that *"Unlike yesterday's leadership requirement for stabilization and grow, today's leaders must transform their organization's values, beliefs, and behaviors."* Representing Forces #1 and #3, the intent of this component is to transform the organization to *"meet the future."* I have serious concerns about organizations transforming their values just to be acceptable to some future vision of change. Remember my concerns regarding medical and nursing education brainwashing reforms being implemented? Well, this is yet another bar in the same music composition!

2) Structural Empowerment. This component is said to represent Forces #2, #4, #10, #12 and #14 and follows the previous by intending to build a *"strong professional*

practice." It also endorses relationships with community organizations to *"improve patients' outcomes."* In general, anything pertaining to this component is simply an operational component of the ideas covered under the previous one.

3) Exemplary Professional Practice. This is considered to be the essence of the MRP, and it is said to entail a *"comprehensive understanding of the role of nursing."* It includes Forces #5, #8, #9, #11 and #13.

4) New Knowledge, Information, & Improvements. This one represents Force #7, which at first sight appears logical. However, once again we find alarming statements that indicate a progressive change. For example, *"our current systems and practices need to be redesigned and redefined..."* Why? We don't even seem to be able to get people to understand the current ones, or for that matter the more traditional and fundamental ones.

5) Empirical Quality Results. This is probably the only component with some logic and sense. It is concerned with outcome analysis and represents Force #6. My concern has to do with how outcomes are assessed, and the historical liability of previous nursing research, which is plagued by pseudoscience.

The most concerning aspect of all of this is the language in which all of these components and forces of magnetism are described. I can only imagine the gallons of Kool-Aid® the writers must have drank in order to spread some much progressive fertilizer. I can assure you that, should you wish to go to the ANCC website and read more about this topic, you should have some Pepto-Bismol® handy so you can counteract the indigestion you are likely to get from the material you will read. However, you are unlikely to read any details about all the money involved in this process, or the troubling aspects of the hurdles any candidate organization must endure in order to earn this designation. As of 2010, there were 372 designated Magnet™ hospitals in our country; their journey to achieving this status taking an average of 4 ¼ years. The cost for this process varies between $100,000 and $600,000 per year and I am very skeptical of its worth. You be the judge!

In summary, nursing leadership is not even remotely similar to what it used to be. At the bedside level the so-called "Nursing Directors" are not the *best of the best*, the way "Head Nurses" used to be. Instead, they are representative of a culture that rewards the accumulation of meaningless academic degrees irrespective of any degree of competence, as well as the endorsement of bureaucracy and committee work as a way of life. Proof of this shift of the priorities of nursing leadership is the proliferation of layers of middle management nursing positions, all of which are geared at increasing the bureaucratic machinery that seems to be necessary in order to operate hospitals nowadays. Within this ethos, nurse managers constitute a relatively young field of endeavor that spawned directly from the creation of managed care. As such, like many other aspects of our downgraded system, these individuals expand the energy expenditure without adding value to patient care. Finally, to make matters worse, there is an entire organizational movement that designates hospitals as Magnets™; organizations that allegedly advance nursing leadership and improve the quality nursing, even though their original purpose was to keep nurses happy irrespective of their competence. Who benefits from this bureaucratic state of affairs? The patients? The nurses? Nah! Just follow the money...

13

Physician Leadership

"Why would I want to join a club that would have me as a member?"

Groucho Marx (Paraphrased)
American Humorist and Movie Star
(1890 - 1977)

As far back as I can remember, when as a child I first expressed my interest in becoming a physician, I thought I would be joining a group of special people; individuals with compassion, integrity, honor, dedication, and a practical measure of altruism. Unfortunately, I was wrong. As it turns out, and at the risk of sounding excessively proverbial, the physician community also includes *"the good, the bad and the ugly"* just like any other subset of our society. From this point of view, it becomes readily apparent that the group that was meant to lead any and all healthcare initiatives is simply not up to doing so, and in general has abdicated its leadership position within the system. Don't believe me? Let's look at the current state of affairs.

Without question, the physician community is the most educated within all of the health professions, and clearly much more than the administrators, researchers, investors, politicians, and every other bureaucrat that plagues the healthcare system. We are, at least for the time being, the only ones with a licensed authority to prescribe medications, order therapy (e.g. physical, respiratory), admit and discharge patients from any hospital, interpret diagnostic tests, and perform therapeutic procedures. You would think that, with all these exclusive attributes, the entire system would revolve around our relationship with the patients, such as I described in Chapter 1 and illustrated in Figure 1–1. However, that is not the case and, in fact, it is precisely this topic that I will describe in the next few pages, to show the degree of downgrading our healthcare system has achieved. Moreover, the breakdown of physician leadership in our country has had many consequences, the most palpable being the progressive overreaching by other groups into the medical scope of practice.

Let's begin by examining the issue of prescribing medications, a responsibility traditionally reserved to physicians. At the present time, there are other parties within the system that are capable of doing so, some with more restrictions than others, and yet some others who continue to seek additional privileges along these lines. For example, both physician's assistants and nurse practitioners (both members of a group known as *physician extenders*) are licensed to prescribe medications, even if they do so under the supervision of "collaborating physicians". To be perfectly clear about my position in this issue, I am not putting down the worthiness of these professionals. I have had the opportunity to "collaborate" with numerous nurse practitioners over the years, many of which have been incredibly capable partners. In fact, at the time of this writing my nurse practitioner has been working with me for over six years (longer than any accredited postgraduate neurology residency program) and I am convinced that she can run circles around most practicing neurologists. That said, the movement that we see across the nation is one in which these individuals continue to be granted increasing independence from physicians either by regulatory changes or simply from the practical point of view. Although this is not necessarily bad, the public must understand that being treated by a physician extender is not quite the same as being treated by the physician himself. In other words, it is impossible to generalize from the experience of one or another group (mine included) to every other physician extender across the land. Consequently, to think that substituting physicians with extenders results in an even trade is not only unreasonable but also unfair to the patients. Nevertheless, the reader should recognize a common thread throughout this book in which I point out how education reform and regulatory legislation provide the underpinnings for a national transformation of the system; a replacement of the traditionally most intellectually sophisticated class of practitioners for a more pliable group of individuals, more likely to follow the mandates of politicians and the *intelligentsia*. For example, in 11 states, nurse practitioners can practice independently and without physician oversight. In this context, the privilege of being able to prescribe medications is progressively being expanded at such a pace that it becomes barely noticeable, even though the ultimate result will be a system in which it will no longer be the sole responsibility of physicians. Finally, following some of my comments about the evolving role of pharmacists pertinent to patient care (Chapter 10), let's just say that having a

"Consultation Window" inside pharmacies (Figure 10-1) is only the beginning. There is absolutely no doubt that pharmacists are very interested in being a source of information for patients relative to medications. The unspoken truth, however, is that there is a dissident movement geared at continuing to expand pharmacists' privileges to prescribe medication internationally. In some countries, including the United Kingdom, Australia, Canada and New Zealand, this is already a reality. In our country, just as there has been a progressive movement at the national political level, that in one way or another intends to transform these United States to a model similar to European countries, the metamorphosis of pharmacy into a prescribing healthcare profession has also begun (Chapter 10).

The issue of prescribing therapy is just an extension of the previous one with a few differences. Undoubtedly, physicians are required to order any therapy that patients are to receive. However, there is increasing demand for freedom of action on the part of various professional therapy societies. When it comes to physical and occupational therapy, for example, there is a growing tendency for the physician to write orders that read simply "evaluate and treat". This type of order effectively confers the therapist *carte blanche* when it comes to treating the patient. But, does it? Not quite. Paradoxically, the next thing that happens is for the therapist to turn around and ask the physician to sign off on whichever *Plan of Care* he thinks is necessary because that is what the law requires. On the physician's side, such ratification is typically accomplished without much deliberation or review. So, Who is in charge? This question will come up over and over again in this chapter, and we will repeatedly point out that it is the physicians' fault that we are in such a state of confusion. Another examples of clinical overreaching by therapists, as we described in Chapter 10, include physical therapists performing nerve conduction studies and electromyograms, occupational therapists using braces to "change" muscle tone, speech therapists applying "cognitive therapy" to neurologic patients, or insisting in testing swallowing function at inappropriate times, and finally, respiratory therapists directing mechanical ventilator protocols.

At this point, it would be fair for the reader to ask, "What does this all have to do with physician leadership?" Well, the truth is that none of the exposed overreaching initiatives could be possible without the physicians' abdication of their own responsibility. I see this on a daily basis and cannot but come to the conclusion that, as a community, we have become not only intellectually lazy but also complacent about what happens to the patients under our care. Such an attitude is palpable every time I see orders such as: *"Start vancomycin and have pharmacy dosing service specify the schedule"*, or *"Start tube feedings and have nutrition services specify the type and schedule"*. If we embrace this type of practice, we have absolutely no moral ground to complain about other groups usurping our role and responsibilities. That said, when considering this subject, it is fair to ask how we got to this point. The justification that I most commonly hear from physicians is that *"I do it because they do a better job than I do"*. Is that so? Did you not take pharmacology and nutrition courses in medical school? Were you not responsible for dosing antibiotics and choosing tube feeding strategies during residency? If the answer is *"No"* to both of these questions, you should probably get your money back because you had a deficient education. Conversely, if the answer to both of these questions is *"Yes"* then the problem is one of laziness, either intellectual or practical; a point that warrants further consideration.

Intellectual laziness is primarily a cultural problem. It stems from the deficiency in the core educational values established by the system, and the educational priorities we discussed in Chapter 4. As we continue to emphasize the need for physicians to follow guidelines, operate via protocols, and conform to regulations, it is only natural that all other attributes that require energy expenditure (e.g. critical thinking) over the course of time will undergo intellectual involution and, in some instances, just pure atrophy. Just as any other aspect of life, doing the right thing when it comes to using our intellect in the practice of medicine, takes deliberate effort and resiliency. The easy path, the one we see most commonly nowadays, is in direct opposition with the essence of medicine. Laziness of a more practical type may just be a simple financial issue. As we discussed in Chapter 7, physicians' compensation is not what it's all cracked up to be! Most of us work harder for a lesser marginal profit and, as a consequence, cutting corners at times becomes a matter of survival. Along these lines, why would anyone want to spend additional time calculating dosages of antibiotics or planning how to tube feed a patient, when either of these two activities will not lead to additional remuneration. A potential counter argument in this discussion is that physicians who are "true leaders" know when to delegate certain responsibilities to all the members of the team. However, I submit that for all the talk about team building, there is no such thing! In reality, the different minions that swarm around patients' bedsides generally interact with each other but hardly ever do they huddle around a physician during rounds as a real team. Do you find this hard to believe? I invite you to look at Figure 13-1, which depicts a sticker placed in each one of our medical charts everyday to document what is referred to as the "Interdisciplinary Team" daily plan of care meeting. The figure is blank but the way it is found in our charts is typically with the signatures of individuals representing nursing, case management, various therapies, clergy, and pharmacy. In all the years that I have been seeing these stickers in our charts, I have never seen a physician's signature in any of them. So you see, the whole concept of the

Patient Name ______________________________

Date _______________ **Time** _______________

Clinical plan of care and barriers to discharge discussed by interdisciplinary team members:

Signature/Department

________________________ / _______________

________________________ / _______________

________________________ / _______________

________________________ / _______________

________________________ / _______________

________________________ / _______________

Figure 13-1
Interdisciplinary Documentation Sticker

team approach is a hoax; the product of a touchy-feely philosophy revolving around the concept that *"There is no 'I' in TEAM!"* As I mentioned in Chapter 4, this misconception that real teams do not have captains has permeated into the educational reforms currently in place in medical schools and, in my opinion, has resulted in physicians being less able leaders. We can argue endlessly the two aspects of this issue. However, the litmus test is represented by the question: Does the delegation of these tasks improve the quality of care? Only if you were to assume that the competence of the individuals who take the place of the physician in performing them (e.g. dosing antibiotics, designing tube feeding strategies) will do so at a level that is nothing but excellent. In my opinion, this is not generally the case and I find those who disagree with me somewhat hypocritical since they are typically the same individuals who support the notion of these *pseudo-teams*.

Another facet of the downgraded status of physician leadership in our country is that which pertains to the regulatory world. This has both a local and a national component. At the local level, for example, physicians are commonly asked to participate in a variety of hospital processes. These are customarily conducted by means of committee meetings, and are meant to address different aspects of the practice of medicine within the confines of the institution in question. Most notably, these committees spend countless hours discussing the best practices to comply with government mandates and regulatory requirements. Typically, physician participation is by invitation and irrespective of personal interest, willingness, or qualifications. In my view, the majority of physicians feel compelled to be part of this process and reluctantly attend the meetings as expected, simply so they are not single out for not being good "team players". Anyone who has attended any of these meetings, and who has been curious enough to look around the facial expressions of the physicians present, is likely to have been the witness of boredom and absent-mindedness. In confidence, many physicians will say that these activities are nothing but an intrusion on their daily schedule, and a waste of their time since the majority of the decisions made by these committees have been prefabricated even before the meeting took place. Perfect examples of this type of phenomenon are illustrated in Chapter 15. Even worse, these committee meetings almost invariably include some of the middle management nurses we introduced in the previous chapter and, as a bonus, one or more members of the administrative elite, all of whom vehemently make a case for the importance of the committee approving one or another new policy, irrespective of logic, reason or consequences.

The national counterpart of the downgrading effect of current physician leadership on our healthcare system relates to organized medicine. We can easily start our discussion with the American Medical Association (AMA). Upon reviewing the history and the charter of this organization, it is eminently clear that it is nothing more than a trade union, not substantially different from the Service Employee International Union (SEIU) or the United Auto Workers (UAW). As such, it suffers from the same problems that these other organizations have, and it behaves not very differently. For example, the AMA restricts entry into the medical profession by virtue of limiting admission into medical schools. Its Council on Medical Education (CME) carries out this type of "filtering" through its process of approving medical schools. Every state medical licensing board requires candidates to have graduated from CME approved schools. Through the years, the CME has exerted its veiled power to restrict medical school entry, one of the most notable occurrences having been in the 1930's during the depression. The most popular justification for this restriction of entry into the medical profession is the intent to raise the standards of quality. However, as others have argued, a critical look at the licensing hurdles formulated by the CME through the years shows how often they had little to do with quality; for example, citizenship and language requirements.

In addition, as we have discussed in Chapters 4 and 7, the AMA and the specialty societies (i.e. the "leaders" of our profession) are directly involved in other downgrading processes such as fixing prices for medical compensation. What are the stakes? Just remember that the AMA earns over $70 Million per year in royalties from licensing the Current Procedural Terminology (CPT) codes essential for billing medical services. That's not small change! Thus, the collusion between the AMA and the specialty societies involved in the price-fixing I described earlier is nothing short of shameful and unbecoming of our once honorable profession.

So, where is the fundamental problem with physician leadership? Is it an ethical deficiency? Or, perhaps a moral one? I like to think that, at least in part there is simply a disconnection between physicians and the environment in which we operate; or possibly a disarray of our priorities. I will try to shed some light into this question by examining how the current system culture affects the fundamental components of leadership. Let's start by emphasizing the importance of culture in leadership. Culture is a complex entity, flowing from learned, shared, tacit and unconscious assumptions on which people based their daily behavior (i.e. "the way we do things around here"). It is deep, broad and stable; it controls individuals and provides predictability. The disconnection is that, with the exemption of individual private practices, politicians and bureaucrats are the ones who have shaped the current culture of healthcare organizations, not practicing physicians! Accordingly, as we will see below, this simple fact creates a situation in which the current culture negatively influences any attempt at physician leadership. Parenthetically, in my own paranoid and contemptuous view of any government intervention, I don't think we have arrived at this point by chance but rather as part of bigger movement that cannot afford real medical leaders; people capable of "rocking the boat!" Now let's examine this conceptual conflict in more detail. Generally speaking, leadership requires for a physician to have a number of attributes, clustered within four domains (Figure 13-2), as follow:

1) Leading one-self. This includes self-awareness, self-management and self-development. These allow

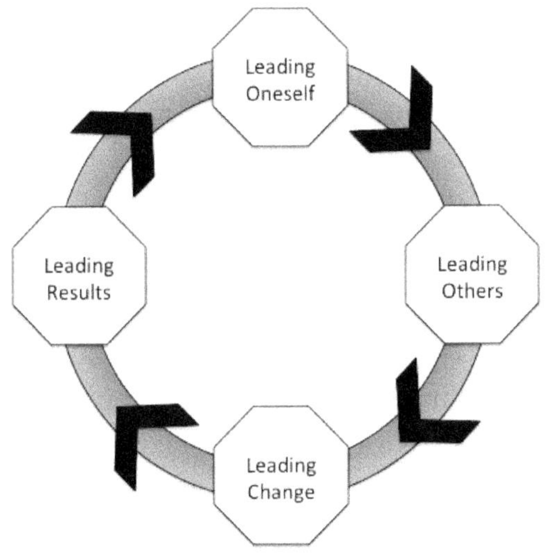

Figure 13-2
Domains of Physician Leadership Effectiveness

physicians to know their strengths and limitations, and take responsibility for personal performance. Although these attributes are largely innate, they require nurturing through proper education. If you remember the discussion in Chapter 4, you should recognize the first downgrading influence.

2) Leading others. Here is where we place the ability to build effective (i.e. real) teams and successfully

communicate a vision or sense of purpose. Our discussion in the previous pages underscores the problem of the current environment being content with pseudo-teams. Yes; another hurdle for effective leadership.

3) Leading change. The ability to manage entire teams and organizations through change takes courage, discipline and persistence. The attributes within this domain are intimately related to those in the previous one, managing change requires a cohesive and effective team.

4) Leading results. This requires a vision of the overall mission, and the ability to make sound decisions.

And so, we see how some of the problems we have already discussed elsewhere in the book interfere with the different attributes required for leadership. The result is a broken down version of the physician as a leader; an ineffective and distorted imitation of the ideal of leadership.

In summary, despite the fact that physicians are the most educated of the "healthcare providers", the last thirty years have seen a progressive erosion of their role as leaders. This aspect of the downgrading process of the healthcare system has taken place due to a variety of factors that include deleterious cultural changes in our society and an increase of the government regulatory control. The latter, at least in view, has not taken place by happenstance but rather as part of a more widespread process that progressively removes the physician as a variable in the leadership equation of the system. However, regardless of causation, it is important for physicians to realize that the core problem is internal rather than external. No one has forced us down the path that takes a group that was originally intended to encompass the best of the best, and lowers the bar to such level that mediocrity becomes a common attribute of our profession. While traditionally physicians were characterized by a passion for excellence, more recently we seem to have embraced a philosophy that could easily be illustrated by an aphorism from W. Somerset Maugham: *"Only the mediocre man is always at his best!"* Until we are willing to look at the mirror in order to find the source of our shortcomings, rather than to look out the window in a feeble attempt at blaming external factors, we will be nothing but complicit instruments of our own demise.

14

Quality and Safety Measures

"In theory there is no difference between theory and practice. In practice, there is."

Yogi Berra
American Hall of Fame Baseball Player and Manager
(1925 - Present)

Quality and safety... Even with a great deal of effort it would be difficult to find two worthier metrics to gauge how successful we are in everyday patient care. Nevertheless, the series of actions instigated by the government and its crony surrogates with the excuse that the current state of affairs in healthcare promotes low quality and unsafe practices, are not of comparable merit. We've already covered some of the ideas pertaining to these interwoven topics in the previous chapters, particularly in our discussions on medical malpractice and the Joint Commission (TJC). Nonetheless, I thought it would be important to specifically address the plethora of initiatives and regulations that are raining on us incessantly from paternalistic government agencies bound and determined to have things their way. The full impact of these activities has yet to be seen and we certainly have not yet seen the bottom of the hole we are digging in order to accommodate centralized control of medical care. I warn you though that my remarks regarding all of these activities, although overly critical and sometimes harsh, do not even begin to paint an accurate picture of the *downgrading* effect they are having, and will continue to have on the medical care we all receive.

Since I have already familiarized the reader with the historical background, organizational structure and operations of TJC, I will start the present discussion by similarly describing the Agency for Healthcare Research and Quality (AHRQ). Formerly known as the Agency for Health Care Policy and Research, the AHRQ is one of 12 agencies within the U.S. Department of Health and Human Services (DHHS), and it is said to be *"dedicated to improving the quality, safety, efficiency, and effectiveness of healthcare for all Americans."* Once again, I have no quarrel with such a lofty goal! However, the real question is whether such a responsibility should lie with the government, or whether it would simply be better to allow the free market to dictate how quality care rises to the top because it is demanded, while unsafe care finds no one to harm because it is not demanded. But oh! I forgot; we do not have a free market in U.S. healthcare, and have not had it for over forty years! In any case, I digress... The AHRQ boasts that it works with both the public and the private sectors and that, in doing so, it *"builds the knowledge base for what works - and does not work - in health and health care and translates this knowledge into everyday practice and policymaking."* If you have been following along the thematic I have introduced so far throughout the book, you will agree with me that the previous statement is code for *"We are going to tell you how to practice medicine!"* Still, it is worthwhile to examine step-by-step the processes that this agency, in collaboration with other organizations (e.g. TJC) and the *medical intelligentsia,* uses to assure quality and safety in everyday practice. It will also be important to discuss the results and unintended consequences of their initiatives and mandates.

However, before we take the plunge into the substance of our discussion, I want to take a moment to bring to your attention a term that you will encounter *ad nauseam* in the pages that follow, and certainly any time you decide to independently read other current sources of information about healthcare. I am referring to the obsessive practice of denoting high quality healthcare as *"Patient-Centered".* This is the latest buzzword; a term introduced by the *medical intelligentsia* and the regulators as if it were a new idea resulting from an epiphany. The champion of the concept of Patient Centered Care (PCC) is the ubiquitous Institute of Medicine (IOM), whose definition of this subject would lead any observer to believe that they just discovered how to boil and egg! No, seriously... Let's just say, for the sake of argument that the brain trust at the IOM had really stumbled into a shiny bright new idea. How should we interpret this? If in the past we have not been practicing PCC, *what is it that we have been doing?* In what have we been "centering" the care we have delivered for so many years? See? Maybe it is not such a new idea after all. That said, as you read on further you will come across the case I make about how what they call PCC is nothing more than superfluous labeling of smoke and mirrors. Moreover, I think I have made it clear how skeptical I am about programs that originate in the government or its surrogates (the IOM being one of the most notorious in our system) and so, I have not been impressed or dissuaded by arguments made under the premise of advancing PCC. Along these lines, and before I forget, let me also point out that the behavior of the IOM as it relates to patient safety, and taking into consideration their data which we analyzed in Chapter 9, has been analogous to that of the political progressive movement at the national level; a behavior crystallized by the current mayor of Chicago and former Chief of Staff of President Obama, Rahm Emanuel: *"You never let a serious crisis go to waste"*. And so, it has been fitting for the IOM to run around, hands in the air, wailing that there is a crisis of errors producing unsafe medical care in order to justify additional policies and regulations. But, enough of that for now! Let's get back to our discussion.

As any other government agency, the AHRQ lists several primary focus areas, as follow:

1) <u>Comparing the Effectiveness of Treatments</u>. AHRQ's patient-centered (here we go!) outcomes research *"Improves healthcare quality by providing patients and physicians with <u>state-of-the-science</u> information on which medical treatments work best for a given condition".* In other words, they compare drugs, medical devices, tests, surgeries, and so on. Well, to begin, this is all very similar to what *Consumer Report* does for other services and products without taxpayers having to foot the bill. But what AHRQ statement does not take into account is the fact that, in medicine, what is good for patient A may not be necessarily good for patient B. Therefore, by disregarding the second domain of Evidence Based Medicine (EBM) we discussed in Chapter 2 (i.e. expert opinion), the AHRQ has turned away from the *Art* of medicine; in fact, notice how they phrase their statement captioned above as "state-of-the-science" rather than the traditional "state-of-the-art". Moreover, the intent on

directly providing patients with information is nothing short of an intrusion in the physician-patient communication flow, and a scheme that is destined to cause more confusion, enhanced mistrust, and negatively impact outcomes.

2) Quality Improvement and Patient Safety. The agency funds and disseminates research geared at identifying root causes of threats to patient safety. Some of its initiatives include preventing healthcare–associated infections, medical liability reform, patient safety culture assessment tools, and more EBM projects designed to improve communication and teamwork skills. Let's look at all of these assertions for a moment. There is no question that finding root causes for threats to patients' safety is a worthwhile proposition. However, the idea that it is reasonable to think that there would be a one-size-fits-all solution that can be shoved down the throat of hospitals and other organizations and forcefully compel them to follow mandates does not sit very well with either my logic or my idea of how government should operate. Likewise, the prevention of infections is also a very reasonable target. However, it is redundant for this agency to engage in activities that are already being covered by TJC. When it comes to medical liability reform, we have already addressed it in Chapter 9, so I will not beleaguer the reader with more on this subject for now. Then there is the development of a patient safety culture; this should stem from the people who make up that culture and their leaders (see my comments about this subject in Chapter 13) and not from external advisors.

3) Health Information Technology. I have some serious problems with this focus area. Let me start by pounding on one of my favorite recurring themes: We do not need information technology for *Health*! If anything, we should be talking about *Medical Information Technology*, since the information being acquired, analyzed, transmitted, and stored is all related to medical care. That said, the agency's goals within this area are stated as: *"Improve healthcare decision-making, support PCC, and improved the quality and safety of medication management."* Interestingly, I find it paradoxical that, on one hand the AHRQ is very interested in empowering patients with information, but has not figured out that even before computers were invented, the patients have always had the power to have an updated list of their medications and other pertinent medical information with them even if they are seen by multiple physicians concurrently. This oversight on their part underscores one of the conflicts between the topics I will discuss in Chapters 18 and 19: *How frequently patients are so busy focusing their attention in information that is not necessary for them to handle, while at the same time they have to be practically forced to bring updated lists of medications with them to clinic!*

4) Prevention and Care Management. It sounds benign enough, doesn't it? The truth is that, as I will discuss at length at the very end of the book, the whole idea of *Preventive Medicine* is a hoax. At least, the way the politicians, bureaucrats and regulators are using it. Suffice it to say though, with the excuse of preventing illness, this agency is bound to introduce initiatives that sometimes are mind-boggling for those of us who live in

the medical trenches and fight disease on a daily basis. Remember how not so long ago the media was on fire about controversial recommendations by a government group to reduce the screening for breast cancer through the use of mammograms, and that for prostate cancer using Prostate Specific Antigen (PSA) testing? Well, guess what? These two recommendations originated from the U.S. Preventive Services Task Force, an independent panel that is part of this focus area of the AHRQ. If this does not sound to you as the government and its cronies inciting a change in medical decision-making, despite opposition from practicing physicians, I don't know what does.

5) Healthcare Value. I spent some time discussing the issue of value as it relates to quality and cost in Chapter 8, but I would like to reiterate that any discussion about value that only relates it to cost is inaccurate, misleading and dishonest. Therefore, in looking at the descriptors used by the AHRQ to describe this focus area I am skeptical about their methodology and by inference, their results and recommendations.

Now that we have covered some of the salient features of the AHRQ, let's combine what we know about this agency with the initiatives introduced by TJC and the Center for Medicare and Medicaid Services (CMS). The most practical way to cover this topic is to begin by reviewing the history of quality measurements in our country. Our journey begins in 1998, when TJC launched its ORYX® initiative. This was the first national program for measuring hospital quality, and originally required non-standardized data of performance measures to be reported. Several years later, in

2002, hospitals accredited by TJC where required to collect and report data on at least two of the so-called *"Core Measures"* (i.e. acute myocardial infarction, heart failure, pneumonia, and pregnancy). From this point on, the collection of data relative to quality has undergone an exponential growth and, as of 2004, the CMS began to penalize hospitals financially if they did not report to them the same data that they were collecting for TJC. This punitive regulatory conduct resulted from TJC and CMS combining their efforts in producing what are now called National Hospital Quality Measures (NHQM). The proliferation of performance measures has been accompanied by public reporting of those measures, as well as by CMS adding data intended to assess patient satisfaction, mortality and readmission due to common medical conditions. More recently, in 2010, TJC began to split its performance measures into two groups: accountability and non-accountability (we presented this topic in Chapter 11). Oddly, after such categorical definition, TJC has been progressively "retiring" its non-accountability measures; doesn't that make you question how important were they in the first place? The bottom line is that the landscape for quality indicators and measures required of hospitals continues to evolve, morph, and grow. As we will see in the next few pages, it is not that some of the indicators do not make sense; they do! The problem is the creation of an incredibly convoluted, bureaucratic and intrusive system of data collection and reporting that does not take into account the individual patient but rather the patient population with a specific illness. I cannot help to ask myself, is this truly patient-centered? As if all of this centralized control of healthcare quality is not enough, other semi-private non-profit (of course!) organizations such as the National Quality Forum

(NQF) and the Hospital Quality Alliance (HQA) have openly endorsed the NHQM. Who makes up these organizations? Anybody who is anybody! The so-called "stakeholders of healthcare"! As you can imagine, having the *de facto* buy-in from every other organized group practically guarantees that the Kool-Aid® flows throughout the entire system.

The core measures whose data are presently required from hospitals across the nation are listed in Table 14-1. Not every one of these applies to every organization and, therefore, I am going to restrict my comments to those that are currently within my immediate practice environment (i.e. those that the hospitals in which I work presently measure).

Acute Myocardial Infarction	Children's Asthma Care
Heart Failure	Surgical Care Improvement Project
Pneumonia	Hospital Outpatient Measures
Perinatal Care	Venous Thromboembolism
Inpatient Psychiatric Services	Stroke

Table 14-1. Core Measures Sets

1) <u>Acute Myocardial Infarction (AMI) Measures</u>. As I noted earlier, I think the indicators within this measure set are fairly reasonable, with one exception. There is no doubt that prompt administration of thrombolytic (i.e. "clot-busting") drug to these patients, as well as performing angioplasty and stent placement when necessary have a direct effect on survival. Furthermore, assuring that upon discharge they are taking aspirin is also very reasonable. In my opinion, however, the data on the use of statins (i.e. a class of medications to improve cholesterol profile) does not take into consideration the quality of life of the patients who take these drugs. This is a subject that I will cover in greater depth in Chapter 20.

2) Heart Failure (HF) Measures. This set of indicators is somewhat puzzling to me. How could anyone have a diagnosis of HF without having undergone some type of evaluation of left ventricular function (i.e. the performance of the heart chamber that pumps blood into the rest of the circulation and whose dysfunction is the hallmark of HF)? And yet this is being tracked by the brain trust! Does anyone really think that this diagnosis could exist without such an evaluation having been performed? In addition, another one of the indicators within this set is common to other core measures: Giving instructions upon discharge. Really? Should not all patients be given instructions upon discharge? Why would we single out this population? Interestingly, the data shows that the patients who receive instructions are less likely to be readmitted for HF. However, not all the instructions within the set carry the same weight and a review of what is being recommended shows an incredible paternalistic attitude towards the patients. Bear in mind that it is the people who want the patients to be "empowered" the ones also championing this approach.

3) Stroke (STK) Measures. These indicators are very dear to me, since they fall smack down into my area of expertise. As such, I have several criticisms relative to their practical application. The first one is a theoretical one: the measures are only applicable to *Ischemic Stroke* (i.e. those that result from a blocked artery with tissue damage from blood flow being cut off) and not to just any stroke. Although at first you may think this is a simple matter of semantics, I can assure you that the hospital

coders and case managers have significant difficulties telling the difference and, therefore, often find deficiencies where there are none. The other major type of stroke, known as *Hemorrhagic Stroke*, results from the rupture of a blood vessel with resulting hemorrhage (i.e. bleeding) in the brain. As you can imagine, the four indicators that require administration of blood thinners do not even apply to these patients. Yet, it is not uncommon to find how these patients are amalgamated with the others in one of the common statistical *maelstroms* we come across in committee meetings. Once we step beyond this philosophical issue, we find more practical ones. If the primary process we are concerned about is one of closure of a blood vessel by a blood clot, why would the government have to bird-dog the utilization of blood thinners in these patients? The reason is that the current *neurologic intelligentsia* has created a mess of this whole topic based upon their distorted view of EBM. As such, the use of blood thinners in patients with ischemic stroke has been made a lot more complicated than it needs to be. The remaining indicators in this set suffer from some of the problems I have discussed elsewhere. The one requiring the use of statins and education upon discharge were covered earlier in the context of AMI. The one on VTE prophylaxis seems redundant and unnecessary unless you ignore the one we're going to discuss next. Then there is the last one; a stroke patient must be assessed for rehabilitation! Wow! If we have to be told by the government that a patient who has a neurologic deficit must be assessed for rehabilitation because we cannot figure that out for ourselves, we should be looking for a different line of work. In a free-market, this is exactly what would happen.

Instead, we are providing safety nets for mediocre practitioners to continue to operate and, in the process, we are shortchanging patients.

4) Venous Thromboembolism (VTE) Measures. This is another set of indicators that largely belongs in what I call *"The Journal of Duh!"* The predisposing factors for VTE have been known for years (even before I became a physician). Why is it that we must continue to micromanage this process in the same way that I mentioned when speaking about the use of blood thinners in patients with ischemic stroke? And then there are... ...more discharge instructions!

5) Pneumonia (PN) Measures. Another set of baffling quality indicators: The government requires for blood cultures to be obtained prior to administration of the appropriate antibiotic. Imagine that! The agencies responsible for this are insisting that we practice Medicine 101! Myself, I take a different position. Strictly speaking, a persistent and consistent pattern of not carrying out these two steps should be grounds for dismissal from the medical staff! But wait! The problem is that the diagnosis of pneumonia is not always very clear from the front end, and yet the assessment by *Big Brother* is done in retrospect. Would you like to know how crazy this makes hospital administrators? I have been in committee meetings and heard an administrator ask a physician, *"Can't you just not go ahead and give the patients a dose of antibiotics before you get a diagnosis so at least we are in compliance?"* And we dare call this quality of care and patient safety!

6) Surgical Care Improvement Project (SCIP) Measures. This set of quality measures is a *mélange* of antibiotic selection prescription and discontinuation, more VTE prophylaxis, and the appropriate treatment of a variety of other perioperative conditions. In general, as I noted earlier, they're all very reasonable goals. My criticism is the same as before: If physicians are not doing this to begin with, where did they get their education? And furthermore, what does their certification and medical licensing then really mean? Do you follow? In any case, perhaps the most distorted aspect of the SCIP measures in general has to do with initiatives regarding *Wrong–site Surgery* (WSS). This term applies to surgical procedures performed on the wrong site of the body, on the wrong side of the body, or in the wrong patient altogether. These cases typically gain national attention via the media and almost invariably result in a malpractice claim that is either settled or paid in full. Their existence, considered part of *Never Events* (a topic that we will discuss the next few pages) and exceedingly rare, has led to procedural changes that require compliance with additional regulations. My question is, does this problem warrant such an overhaul of the system or are we again barking up the wrong tree? In the first place, the estimated incidence of WSS is 1 in 113,000 or so operations. If we apply some of the rules we discussed in Chapter 9, this numbers yield approximately 8.9 defects per million (DPM) opportunities and places to historical data at almost Six-Sigma (6σ) levels (Figure 9-1); and this is without anyone moving a muscle to improve the system! Instead, site verification protocols have been implemented all over the nation and have been monitored by the regulatory agencies. Interestingly, the

data available in the literature emphasize that these protocols *could have prevented* about 2/3 of the cases only, and point out how their complexity does not relate to any value-added.

In addition, just as we noted earlier, CMS and AHRQ have added their own sets of measures, as follow:

1) Mortality Measures (CMS)

2) Patients' Experience of Care Measures (CMS)

3) Readmission Measures (CMS)

4) Patient Safety Indicators (PSI) Composite Measures (AHRQ)

5) PSI and Nursing Sensitive Care.

6) Healthcare–Associated Infections Measures.

7) Global Immunization (IMM) Measures.

8) Emergency Department (ED) Throughput Measures.

I will not beleaguer the reader further by describing my objections to each one of these since they are, after all, secondary. However, several points deserve mention. For example, by what equation does ED *throughput* relate to quality? In Chapter 16, we discussed the current state of affairs relative to medical emergencies, it will be clear that there are numerous variables that affect the passage of one patient through the ED. Moreover, it does not really matter that a patient has not yet left ED to be placed in his assigned nursing unit bed, if definitive treatment has already been started.

Another set of indicators that does not seem to be related to quality of care in the strict sense of the word is that entitled *"Patients' Experience of Care"*. In my view, this is the federal equivalent of the obtuse "Patient Satisfaction Scores" hospitals continue to analyze as a measure how successful they are. It is in fact at the core of the transformation of hospitals from a medical service to a hospitality industry! Don't believe me? The next time you're in the hospital you will see how the people who bring food are now referred to as "Room Service", just as they would be in a hotel. The beds are set in the same as those you find in a Hilton or a Marriott. In the past, I have been openly critical (imagine that!) of how hospitals congratulate themselves on achieving "95% Satisfaction Scores" when they have sampled less than 5% of the admissions for the study period; it is comical how they ignore fundamental statistical rules of sample size calculation. To make matters worse, treating patients from this point of view encourages the entitlement behavior we will discuss in Chapter 18.

Readmission measures also need to be addressed specifically. If nothing else because the current mentality is that if a patient gets readmitted with the same diagnosis that led to his recent discharge, someone must not be doing his job! Alas, this may or may not be the case since many illnesses by their own nature result in recurrent admissions due to the fact that they have an inherent instability. One of the reasons this is important is because HF is one of those. Yes, as we said earlier, it may be possible to decrease this rate by educating the patient but there are changes beyond the control of either the treatment team or the patient himself that may lead to unwanted readmissions. The alarming aspect of this topic is the fact that the Affordable Care Act (ACA) (i.e. Obamacare) already includes provisions by which CMS will cut down payments to hospitals with "relatively high" readmission rates.

And then there is the issue of infections secondary to healthcare experiences, particularly those related to intravenous catheters, or to indwelling bladder catheters. It has been my experience that in both of these scenarios, there are two major opportunities: a) Placement of the device, and b) Its subsequent care. The former requires for the individual placing it to adhere to strict guidelines of sterility. If I had a penny for every time I have seen this dictum breached, I probably would not even need to worry about whether this book sells or not. The solution for the intravenous catheters placed in central veins (i.e. the large veins around the chest area) is the use of what is known as a "maximal sterile barrier" technique. There is absolutely no excuse for not following such a procedure in 2012. But, is this a recent model? Not at all! As early as 1991, we were already routinely using this practice. The placement of indwelling bladder catheters also requires a sterile technique on the part of the nurses who are the ones typically carrying this out. Unfortunately, as we mentioned in Chapter 5, nursing education is currently more concerned with issues of "social justice" than teaching bedside nurses how to carry out tasks optimally; the hospitals' solution to this problem? Teams of two nurses, one of which confirms that the other one's method of placing the catheter has met all requirements. Now, there's an idea; *one questionably competent individual supervising another!* The subsequent care of both intravenous and bladder catheters is strictly a nursing issue. In their defense, if we continue to prioritize their time in filling out forms that fulfill compliance regulations, their attention will be diverted from important tasks such as caring for catheters to prevent them from getting infected. It is important to recognize that the indicator relative to infections of indwelling bladder catheters is also part of an initiative by TJC known as the National Patient Safety Goals (NPSG), introduced in 2002. I mentioned this for the sake of completeness because, in my opinion, the NPSG has significant redundancy with every other organization we have discussed earlier.

Also in 2002, the NQF published a report entitled *"Serious Reportable Events in Healthcare: A Consensus Report 2"*, in which it listed 27 different adverse events (AE) that were *"serious, largely preventable and of concern to both the public and healthcare providers"*. As a group, these became known as *"Never Events"*, with the implication that none of them should ever take place in a hospital. These *Never Events* were grouped into several categories:

1) <u>Surgical or Invasive Procedure Events</u> (e.g. surgery performed on the wrong site; objects left inside patient).

2) <u>Product or Device Events</u> (e.g. intravascular air embolism).

3) <u>Patient Protection Events</u> (e.g. injury from patient elopement; suicide).

4) <u>Care Management Events</u> (e.g. unsafe administration of blood products; injury from a fall; stage 3 &4 pressure ulcers).

5) Environmental Events (e.g. injury from physical restraint or bed ails).

6) Radiologic Events (e.g. injury from a metallic object within the MRI area).

7) Potential Criminal Events (E.g. physical abuse).

It was not long after this that CMS began to introduce the concept of *"Pay for Performance"* (P4P) in an attempt to hold hospitals accountable by linking reimbursement to behavior. This idea led CMS in 2008 to introduce a new policy by which it would not pay for any cost associated with the following Never Events: a) Pressure ulcer stages 3& 4, b) Falls and trauma, c) Surgical site infections after certain procedures, d) Infections of intravenous catheters, e) Infections of indwelling bladder catheters, f) Administration of incompatible blood, g) Air embolism, and h) Objects left unintentionally after surgery.

So far, we have limited our discussion to government intervention to "promote quality and safety" in hospitals across our nation. But what about the outpatient practices many of us have? The latest intrusion into our professional lives with the excuse that "government knows best" is a project called *"Meaningful Use"* (MU). The American Recovery and Reinvestment Act of 2009 (ARRA), also known as the "stimulus bill", included funds to be spent in providing incentives (or bribes if you will) to providers and facilities that demonstrate their MU of electronic medical records (EMR). Make no mistake, I have been a supporter of the use of EMR from the very beginning; in fact, having designed and programmed some forms of EMR for the use of my team while I was still at the University. Over the course of the years, I have studied, sampled, and used different EMR products in my daily practice. I found all of them to invariably be inadequate from one point of view or another, requiring an enormous amount of effort in time and energy on my part to tweak them to suit their practical use in medicine. Therefore, I think I have sufficient perspective and justification to state without an ounce of doubt that the MU initiative on the part of the government is absolutely a scam. It is nothing more than government telling us how to practice and how to collect information that is clinically meaningless; for example "ethnicity". Frankly, it also concerns me the large amount of personal data that will be available to Big Brother to be used at his whim. In any case, the way it works is that CMS pays extra monies once it is documented that the practitioner is complying with the requirements of MU. I will expand further in Chapter 23.

In summary, quality of care and patient safety are worthwhile goals. Vigilance on the part of physicians, hospitals and anyone else involved in the delivery of patient care is not only appropriate but also necessary. However, the extraordinarily complex, redundant, and bureaucratic system created by the government (i.e. CMS, DHHS, AHRQ) and its surrogates (i.e. TJC, NQF, IOM) cannot be completely justified and must be viewed as a collusion of those in the elite echelons of the healthcare system to impulse centralized control of the delivery of care. At the risk of sounding paranoid again, the fact that these agencies have popularized the existence of a "medical error crisis" based on a small proportion of the ongoing medical encounters, just so they can intervene by means of their policies, is alarming. It is also suggestive that their ultimate goal is to shift the control of patient care to bureaucratic committees that will issue edicts with the expectation of universal compliance. This idea is already manifested in the Independent Payment Advisory Board (IPAB) of the ACA; a group of 15 unelected officials who eventually determine which practices will be covered and which ones will not. Do we need a systematic approach to quality of care and patient safety? Indeed we do! However, I submit that it is irrelevant for medical schools to have such strict criteria for accepting new students, and for certification and licensing boards to make it so difficult to gain their endorsement, if at the end of the day it would be the government bureaucrats and their cronies who are going to be looking over our shoulder on a daily basis to see if we practice medicine at the level they think is optimal. Still, in following my discussion in Chapter 4, it is also likely that the reforms to which medical education is being subjected are geared towards producing a public servant that will follow blindly the regulations imposed by those who sit in ivory towers.

15

Hospital Protocols & Policies

"If there are two or more ways to do something, and one of those ways can result in a catastrophe, then someone will do it. (Corollary 18 to Murphy's Law)"

Edward A. Murphy, Jr.
American Aerospace Engineer
(1918 - 1990)

The downgrading process of our medical system could not have had a better tool than hospital protocols and policies. These are sets of pre-packaged ordinances that are intended to serve a specific purpose, either clinical or cultural. They are a component of the ever growing culture of "cookbook medicine" reinforced by the government, its cronies, the bureaucrats and, of course, the intellectually lazy that follow the *medical intelligentsia* without question or query. The hospital leadership committees that we described elsewhere in the book are most commonly responsible for the creation of these protocols. As such, they habitually suffer all the problems of any product of a committee (remember that the definition of a committee is a group of people who set out to design a horse, but ended up with a camel). Committees' lines of sight are so short that they invariably fail to critically assess the root cause of the problem being "solved", or to carefully consider the unintended consequences of the decisions made. The results are consistently disastrous, leading to additional waste of energy, cumulative paperwork, congratulatory statements between the uncritical Kool-Aid®-drinking middle managers, and nothing but additional misery at the bedside. Likewise, even from the get go, the intended beneficial effect of these protocols is, at best, suspect.

At present, hospital protocols and policies abound in any hospital. In my experience, they obey two different motivating sources: a) Some government mandate relative to the Centers for Medicare and Medicaid (CMS) or The Joint Commission (TJC) forcing their agenda on patient safety or their version of quality of care, or b) Peer pressure from fashionable practices initiated by the *medical* and the *nursing intelligentsia*, and followed by hospitals like blind sheep without any inkling of sovereignty, character, or creativity. In both instances, the background data (sometimes carelessly referred to as "research" or even "evidence") are nothing but an amalgamation of poorly constructed hypotheses, biased or incompetent methods, and asinine conclusions. In the case of the government-initiated protocols, there is hardly any debate about the topics at the hospital level, since the recommendations descend on us like manna graciously given to us by "authoritative" panels [e.g. the Institute of Medicine (IOM)]. I thought it would be best to discuss these in the context of their own regulatory processes and, therefore, I direct the reader to our expositions in Chapters 11 and 14.

However, those initiated at the hospital level deserve their own discussion, and this is it!

At the time of this writing, almost every week I come to the hospital to find that a new "protocol" or "policy" has been put in place, the overwhelming majority of them having so many flaws that it makes it almost impossible to execute them without completely ignoring fundamental rules of good medical practice. I have chosen to begin our discussion about this topic around two of the most downgrading protocols or policies.

Intensive Care Open Visitation

Anyone who has either worked or consulted in an intensive care unit (ICU) understands that the critical aspect of this environment, what makes it "intensive", is the obsessive nursing care these patients must receive. The physicians' presence is generally limited to a number of minutes per day at each bedside while making rounds. The way it is supposed to work is that, during this rounding time, the data that the nurses have collected since the last time rounds were made are reviewed, the patient is assessed, opinions from other members of the team are requested (provided there is a "real" team; see Chapters 4 and 13), treatment decisions are made and orders are written. Thus, in any intensive care unit of ten beds, it is possible to make rounds and carry all these tasks in approximately two hours. So, what happens to these patients during the remaining 22 hours of the day? Well, the answer is actually quite simple: *This is the time required to deliver intensive care!* In other words, it is during those other 22 hours that nurses, therapists, pharmacists, and nutritionists are supposed to implement the decisions made by the physician while they concurrently collect additional information to support the decisions that will be made in the next set of rounds. In this context, the reader must understand that the outcome of critically ill patient largely depends on all of these individuals spending time at the bedside *looking after the patient.* Precious time that is necessary to collect numerous pieces of information required to make additional clinical decisions, and to implement the treatment strategies that can lead to the improvement of the patient. Therefore, it is easy to conclude that the term "Intensive Care" is nothing but a contraction of *Intensive Nursing Care Over Time.*

Once we appreciate the premise of this type of clinical environment, it follows that anything that interferes with the intensive contact between nurses (as well as other staff members) and the critically ill patients has the capability of influencing their outcome in a negative way. In the past, the biggest challenge we faced was to make the intensive care nurses understand the importance of such a formula. In fact, any experienced intensive care nurse is likely to agree that it would be practically impossible to improve the clinical status of these patients without paying very close attention to the moment-to-moment changes that take place, and effecting adjustments in treatment to each one of these changes. Anyone who has faced the daunting task of keeping a patient on multiple intravenous drips, ventilatory support, nutritional support, while constantly monitoring labile vital signs, knows exactly the amount of energy and attention that it takes to carry this out. Based upon this philosophy, the traditional view has been that visitors should be allowed for very short periods of time and only when the nurses think the patient is stable enough to tolerate some degree of distraction on her part. This is, in fact, the type of schedule that most of us have been used to, and that worked so well for so many years. Typically, the visitors would be allowed two at a time, for periods between 15 and 30 minutes, and only when the bedside nurse was prepared for them to be at the bedside, usually 4 to 6 times in any 24-hour period. Such a schedule assured that the patients could be visited by their family members; that the latter would be there to provide a comforting voice or a soothing touch to a patient that otherwise would likely not be able to communicate well, but more importantly, that the continuity of the care of the individual would not be jeopardized by any unwanted distractions.

Unfortunately, the changes in priorities we have discussed elsewhere in the book, particularly those related to the preferment of "patient satisfaction", and in this case its surrogate "patient's family satisfaction", as the yardstick for measuring success, have helped create major changes in how we approach the intensive care unit environments. Over the last few years, one of the cultural changes that have been practically shoved down our throats by hospital administrations is that which revolves around *"Open Visitation"*. The theory, introduced by the uncritical thinkers who publish in second or third rate nursing journals and embraced by the *nursing intelligentsia*, is that somehow having visitors and family members all the time in the intensive care unit is beneficial. To this end, hospital policies have been changed against the will of both intensive care physicians and nurses to satisfy the misguided desire of patients families to exercise their "right" to be present at all times, while treatment decisions are being made or therapeutic maneuvers are being executed. The results have been nothing but dreadful, but who cares? Hospital administrators have made it clear that it doesn't really matter what the clinicians think, so long as they get good scores in their patient satisfaction surveys! Just as I have mentioned elsewhere in the book, the most important priority seems to be to keep families happy, not the positive outcome of the patient. In fact, a cursory review of the literature on the subject shows yet one very interesting metric of success: *Decreased complaints!* Well, guess who typically gets to listen to families complain? Administrators! And this is where the rubber hits the road. This whole cultural change is about keeping families out of the

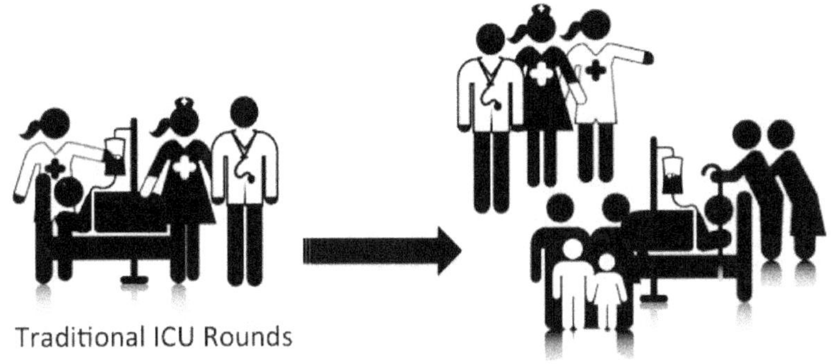

Figure 15–1
The Effect of Open Visitation on Rounds

administrative offices of the hospitals with their selfish complaints!

I think it is important, before the reader thinks that I am callous or that I do not really care about the well being of the family, that I describe what we now have to go through on a daily basis in order to practice intensive care medicine (Figure 15-1). It used to be that we would time our rounds so not to conflict with the short and periodic visitation times the families had. We would arrive at each bedside, and the intensive care nurse working on each particular patient would provide us the flowchart with the data and the medical record. We would then review the data, while the nurse described the salient features of the patient's evolution over the last 12–24 hours, and then proceeded to assess the patient, while reviewing the various monitoring instruments at the bedside. This was also our opportunity to discuss any additional issues with other members of the team present in the intensive care unit. Based upon this broad look at the patient's situation, we would then write our daily notes and the next set of orders relative to the patient's treatment for the next 12-24 hours. We would then move to the next patient and the process would be repeated. Once we had covered all of the patients in the intensive care unit, with a few exceptional situations, we would then go to the waiting area and discuss each patient with his family, providing a summary of the present status and the plan of care for the next interval of 12-24 hours. We would then answer their questions and would go about the rest of our hospital business. The process was structured, predictable, organized and, amazingly "patient-centered"; a term that by now the reader should recognize as one that ironically is very popular among the healthcare bureaucrats and regulators.

At the present time, however, the situation is very different (Figure 15-1). Any time we arrive at the bedside, almost irrespective of the hour of day, there's bound to be someone from the family or simply a visitor in the room with the patient. Many times there are more than one and, in my experience, the average is two. Typically, the moment they see us approach the room where the patient is, they move to intercept us and begin asking questions. Other times, they don't say much but they stand next to us while we're looking at the clinical data, essentially reading over our shoulder. In my practice, a particularly irritating example of the latter behavior took place the other day, when a family member stood next to me while I reviewed the last 24 hour recording of a video electroencephalogram (i.e. continuous brain wave assessment) of the patient, and had the audacity to point at the screen to indicate to me the waves he was sure were "abnormal". Unfortunately this is not an isolated incident. We are the targets of similar unsolicited "diagnostic" commentaries almost daily and about every other monitoring device in the room. How should we respond to such presumptuous, inappropriate and impertinent acts? We do what we can, but the fact is that the problem does not end there; the ubiquitous visitors change tactics on the fly!

So, after going through the disagreeable experience of having to tell an adult that is rapidly firing questions at us to wait until we are finished assessing the patient, we have to endure the fact that they retreat back to the bedside, only to interfere again while we are in the process of evaluating the patient. Such interference can take various forms, the most common of which is answering every time we ask the patient (or the staff) a question or prompting the patient to answer a question that we have asked. Let me illustrate this point with another anecdotal example:

PHYSICIAN: *"Mr. Patient, can you hear me?"*

WIFE: *"Honey, the doctor is here, answer him!"*

PHYSICIAN: *"Mrs. Patient, please..."*

WIFE: *"Oh! Sorry..."*

PHYSICIAN: *"Ms. Nurse, has Mr. Patient been responding over the last few hours?"*

WIFE: *"He responds when I speak to him!"*

At this point, it becomes downright embarrassing to be forced to tell an adult to back off and it is almost impossible to keep one's cool demeanor.

I wish I could say that this is as far as it goes, but it isn't. After we have managed to pushed them out of the way, making sure we don't trample them while approaching the bedside, and have succeeded to somehow complete our assessment of all of the data as described above, we then have to discuss all of our decisions with a group of people that are fascinated by all of the multicolored blinking lights and the numbers in the screens near the patient. Therefore, we have to listen to questions that have absolutely no relevance to the big picture of the patient's clinical condition because they feel the need to understand the causes for a certain digital reading to fluctuate, and the best course of action that we propose to bring it to "normal". In intensive care, this type of explanation can become a daunting task, particularly when multiple family members gang up on you asking questions simultaneously.

In all fairness, the majority of family members who behave this way are aided by two groups of people. The first involves some members of the staff who think it is polite to provide explanations to every single detail of the patient's care since the families are present for every second of every minute they are there themselves. I suspect, although I cannot prove it, that this behavior is the result of a desire to be heard, to have an opinion, to "contribute", or simply the product of an insecure identity. The reader will recall that this was one of the issues I brought up in the first chapter of the book when I discussed how often the "Allied Health Professions" became a hurdle for the basic relationship between the patient and his physician. This is in fact one of the most tangible examples of such a problem.

The second group that influences the behavior of the ICU families in regards to questioning the care the patient is receiving is the one that I call *"The Advisors"*. In order to qualify to be a member of this group, you typically have to be cousin, a neighbor, a coworker, or simply the friend of a friend. Any of these individuals, whom I will further describe in Chapter 19, typically counsels the family from a conceited point of view, suggesting diagnostic and therapeutics alternatives for our patient with authority derived from time spent surfing through *WebMD*, or from having watched countless episodes of *Grey's Anatomy* or *House*. Some close friends of mine refer to these people as *Faux MDs* (*FMD*, for short). The point is that, from afar, these FMDs give the appearance to know medical concepts that the bedside team does not know, and insist that families ask questions to satisfy *their own* inquisitiveness about information they consider crucial; they want us to know that we are not dealing with ignorant people; that we cannot "fool" them by not addressing their "valid" concerns; that we are not the only ones with a "point of view" about the patient's clinical status. Really? Let me share a secret with you: *We are not impressed by FMDs!* Moreover, we find this behavior arrogant, vain, disruptive and distracting!

The truth is that the amount of data we manage in critically ill patients is enormous. In order for any one of these data points to make sense, it must be examined in the context of every other concurrent piece of information. The ability to integrate all of these, as I have discussed before, is one of the primordial characteristics of a physician; one that is polished by the accumulation of knowledge, as well as by the years of experience. To think that a casual visitor in any ICU has the same capability is ludicrous! It follows that, one of our responsibilities when it comes to communicating with families is to "package" all that we know about the patient into relevant statements that are neither unfairly succinct nor confusingly verbose; this also takes experience. I will cover this point at greater length in Chapter 19, but suffice it to say, the last thing we need is for families to demand that we explain why is it that the *pulsatility* of an arterial waveform has changed over the last 12 hours! Especially because the well-meaning cousin insists that this information must be shared. If the reader does not know the meaning of the term *pulsatility*, I just made my point! Alas, the more time families spend at the bedside in the ICU, the more they tend to accrue irrelevant questions.

A final note about Open Visitation policies has to do with privacy and confidentiality. Although this topic will be primarily addressed in Chapter 23, it seems paradoxical that we are compelled by the federal government to a high-priority emphasis on this "patient right", but then we turn around and transform ICUs into train stations, where non-medical personnel walk in and out at will, unescorted, and free to wander around. Believe me, they wander around! The champions of Open Visitation will tell you that part of the policy is for nurses to curb this behavior but, in my view, not only this is not in their job description, but it distracts them from their bedside duties. In any case, it used to be that every nursing unit in a hospital had a board with the last names of the patients and their room numbers for quick reference. After the introduction of the Health Insurance Portability and Accountability Act (HIPAA), however, all of these boards had to be taken down to "protect the privacy" of every Mr. Jones or Mrs. Smith in the hospital. Curiously, the ICU squatters we are discussing are commonly within an earshot of all type of conversations about other patients, and are witness to all sorts of scenes that breach confidentiality at numerous levels. Also ironically, most ICUs also have boards with names that are quite visible to anyone within the premises. So, is this a double standard? Personally, I think this is a predictable consequence of administrators making policy on clinical processes they know nothing about, simply to conform to current uncritical trends, or so they do not have to deal with the self-centered behavior of certain families. To make matters worse, even though I have chosen to discuss this cultural change in the context of ICUs, a similar "open door" policy in in effect in our Emergency Department (ED), making it a wholly unsafe and somewhat chaotic environment. But, enough of beating on a dead horse... Now, let's shift gears and discuss one of my *favorite* hospital protocols.

Rapid Response Team

I remember the meeting as if it were yesterday, even though it took place several years ago. We had been seating around a large table during lunchtime to discuss issues relevant to critical care medicine in our hospital. I was encouraged by having this forum because the committee in which I was sitting at that moment did not exist upon my arrival to this hospital following my departure from the University. Having worked within the ethos of critical care medicine for over two decades had made me realize that the decisions pertinent to this field of medicine were best made by individuals who spent most of their time inside ICUs.

Therefore, as soon as I arrived to this hospital in my new venture, I championed the formation of such a committee. Little did I know that the day in question would be the last time I would attend one of its meetings.

The topic at hand was the poor outcome of patients who required advanced cardiac life support (ACLS) for resuscitation following one or another form of cardiopulmonary arrest. For the reader who may not be familiar with this concept, it is the familiar *"Code Blue"* of movies and television shows. Similarly to what is portrayed in the screen, once such an alarm is triggered, a frantic display of human activity follows, all geared at rescuing some poor soul from a life-threatening cardiopulmonary event. In reality, the majority of these situations end up in unsuccessful outcomes and the patients die. This is not necessarily anyone's fault, although an argument was being made (one with which I happened to agree) that many of these patients did not have to reach the critical point of requiring ACLS if early warning signs were properly identified and corrected.

This was not my first time considering this problem, as I had been the Chair of the Resuscitation Committee at the University Hospital for almost eight years, and the existing literature wholly supported the potential predictability of these catastrophes. However, my own opinion was that the deficiencies in identifying early warning signs of cardiopulmonary crises were closely tied to the downgrading of nursing care, which I have addressed in other chapters. The reader should not have any difficulty relating to this problem since it is a simple matter of common sense. If you take the nursing staff and: a) Dilute their education, b) Exempt them from accountability, c) Shift their priorities from patient care to patient satisfaction, and d) Provide them with *1001 Arabian* forms to fill on a daily basis, it should not be surprising that they are largely incapable of proactively addressing downward trends in patients' clinical status. Once we come to terms with this reality, the most reasonable solution is simple: *Undo all of the above!*

However, that makes too much sense for a group of bureaucrats devoid of critical thinking and eager to please their administrative masters by following like sheep the downgrading trends promoted by the *nursing intelligentsia*. Thus, we were asked on that fateful meeting to consider and approve the creation of *"Rapid Response Teams"* (RRT). According to the middle-management crony who presented this idea, it was one of the most popular concepts being advanced in the nursing community everywhere. Mind you that, as I have expressed elsewhere in the book, the overwhelming majority of individuals at this administrative level do not have the critical thinking skills or scientific experience to distinguish between reliable and unreliable sources of information, or between solid research and pseudoscientific babbling. And so, the explanation that followed described the basic premise of their plan: *To designate, for every shift, specific nurses working in different intensive care units to respond together with a respiratory therapist to the bedside of any nurse that summoned them as an RRT*. Such a team would have the responsibility to "assess" the patient and decide if any immediate testing was necessary (e.g. laboratory studies, arterial blood gases), and carry it out. They were then charged with the responsibility to notify the attending physician of the results of these tests and obtain any orders the physician would give them regarding treatment of the patient. Wow!

Once the awe of all of the other nursing members of the committee had partially subsided, and their mutual congratulatory expressions had been exchanged, the flaw in the entire theory became flagrantly evident to those of us that had been brooding on this problem much earlier than that particular day: Their solution was a *bona fide* Band-Aid! Curiously, and unlike most other times, I was not the first to volunteer to express my skepticism for such a solution. One of my colleagues, a very well respected and experienced pulmonary and critical care specialist, quickly and decisively pointed out that the strategy suggested did not address the core problem of nursing competence at the bedside; it simply shifted the responsibility to other nurses! Several of us lined behind him to suggest that the RRT idea was no different than the biblical metaphor of *"the blind leading the blind"*.

We then proceeded to point out, one at a time, the numerous problems and unintended consequences that would come from implementing this type of policy. Our objections included the dangerous assumption that the nurses to be appointed to these teams were sufficiently knowledgeable and experienced to "assess" patients correctly, and choose the correct diagnostic strategy. The price to pay for such an assumption being wrong was a delay in the definitive care that the patient needed to receive by virtue of circumventing the attending physician, the ultimate decision-maker in each case. My comments were based upon having witnessed the numerous deficiencies that plague bedside nursing, regardless of whether it is in a regular nursing unit or an ICU. Another explicit consequence of the policy being suggested was that the typical bedside nurse would have absolutely no motivation to think critically about any patient who is changing in clinical status because she would not be held accountable due to the fact that she can always call the RRT (Figure 12-1).

After all of us had expressed our skeptical opinions about the proposal, the conversation was summarized by a higher-level administrator in such a way that anyone who had not been present up to that moment, would have thought that everyone of us was in favor of the proposal. Although this led all of us to look at each other in puzzlement, the final blow came later: Less than 72 hours following that meeting, there were full-color posters all over the hospital announcing the creation of RRTs. This could only mean one thing: *The decision to create these teams had already been made prior to our meeting, and all they wanted was a rubberstamp from our committee!* That is when I decided not to continue to waste my time by attending its meetings.

In order to place in perspective my previous comments, let me view the history of RRT, from conception, through maturation and current knowledge. If nothing else, I would like to use this topic as an example of my criticisms of Evidence Based Medicine (EBM) as it is currently applied (see Chapter 2); how people who insist in using the term EBM in every other sentence actually fail miserably at adhering to the evidence. The concept of RRTs, or Medical Emergency Response Teams (MERT) as they are also known, was introduced in the mid 1990's by a group of Australian investigators working in a teaching hospital in order to preempt cardiopulmonary arrests that could be prevented. Again, a hypothesis with which I wholeheartedly agree! However, I would like to emphasize the particulars of their reported experience because they are so different than the current RRTs being used everywhere. In the first place, their concept of MERT was that of a group of *"medical and nursing staff trained in the principles of resuscitation"*, not just a nurse and a respiratory therapist. Furthermore, their medical center was a *"375-bed teaching hospital"* in an urban community, and not just any small private hospital. Immediately, anyone with experience will see where I'm going with this; teaching hospitals in our country have resident physicians in-house all the time, while private community hospitals only have certain physicians available 24/7 (e.g. anesthesiologists, emergency physicians). After collecting data for one whole year, the founders of the concept of MERT (or RRT for that) reported that 70% of all of the calls received for this new team originated in either the ED (62%) or the ICUs (29%). This is a very puzzling finding since it raises some intriguing questions: Why would it be necessary to call an external team to areas of the hospital that should already have personnel conversant with resuscitation? Unless their ED does not regularly staff emergency physicians, why would the MERT be needed to provide care for patients in this area? In regards to being called from ICUs, wasn't the whole point of having an MERT that of transferring certain patients from a regular ward to an ICU bed preemptively? The answers to these questions, one way or another, indicate that neither the hospital environment nor the original design of the team were even remotely similar to what had been discussed with us as a plan for our own hospital; or, where they?

Faced with the quandary of how to reconcile the conceptual differences I have pointed out, one could argue that a single report (even if it is the original one) the body of literature does not make! Unfortunately, anyone who has followed the historical evolution of RRTs by perusing the published reports will quickly realize that it is not the exception but rather the rule that the bulk of the experience with mature RRTs derives from large teaching hospitals, using teams led by physicians (in some cases senior faculty members)! Furthermore, the whole subject brings to mind

Winston Churchill, who once said: *"However beautiful the strategy, you should occasionally look at the results!"* And so, we find that, after all these years, and all the rhetoric about RRTs, the evidence about their effectiveness is... Wait! There isn't any! What? Were our skeptical and dissident opinions during that committee meeting correct? I will let you be the judge of that!

As it turns out, from the very beginning the whole utility of RRTs has been suspect. In the initial 1995 Australian study, for example, their MERT *"superseded the existing cardiac arrest team"*, rather than duplicating it. Therefore, it is not surprising that a large percentage of their calls (28%) were due to *cardiac arrest!* Uhmm.... ...Wasn't this condition the one the MERT was supposed to prevent in the first place? Absolutely! So it seems we have been talking about the proverbial apples and oranges. This is an important point, for it impresses how critical it is to look at the details when reviewing the literature in order to be sure what type of team is being discussed. One of the most experienced of these teams (i.e. University of Pittsburgh), for example, encompasses eight members led by an ICU physician; this MERT does not respond to the ED or to ICUs. In 2004, they reported that their efforts lowered the incidence of cardiopulmonary arrest from 6.5 to 5.4 per 1000 admissions, and they found this to be "statistically significant". Really? You do the Math! That is the same as saying that the MERT lowered cardiopulmonary arrests from 0.65% to 0.54%! Wow! Are you impressed? I am certainly not! Do you remember in Chapter 2 when I mentioned how the use of statistics can be misleading? Well, there you have it! But this is not all; the largest randomized prospective multicenter study (i.e. the "best of the best" in EBM) on the subject, which included over 125,000 patients failed to show a significant reduction in cardiac arrests by RRTs.

Despite the overwhelming evidence, we still live with our RRT and its dysfunctional behavior. In my own personal experience, every single time our RRT has been summoned to the bedside of one of my patients (over all my objections), the unequivocal result has included the performance of unnecessary tests (e.g. measuring blood gases in a patient with clearly evident respiratory embarrassment) and the delay in the administration of definitive therapy which can only occur after I have been contacted. To add insult to injury, there is now a number handed to patients and family members so they can summon the RRT themselves! I will bet you that, if you were to ask any of the RRT devotees, he would tell you that this done so they can be "empowered"! With all due respect, all I have in response to this a term of *agricultural skepticism*.

I think is fair, before I leave the subject, that I give you my own perspective of a more positive alternative method for the problem. Let me start by saying again that I am convinced that a number of cardiopulmonary events may be preempted (not necessarily prevented) using the correct strategy. This requires two components: a) Early recognition and discrimination of impending crises, and b) Decisive delivery of definitive care. The former depends on competent bedside nurses; nothing else will do! As I said earlier, it will be impossible to have a competent nursing body unless we unburden it from all of the bureaucratic tasks they are required to complete, hold them accountable, and support them through education. However, the most recent tactic pertaining to this topic has been exactly the opposite: *To further dumb them down!* The latest achievement of the nursing brain trust has been the introduction of the Modified

Early Warning Score (MEWS) system (Figure 15-2). This is a scale that directs nurses to automatically summon the RRT based upon a patient's score, without having to think! Yes, I was just as puzzled as you probably are right now. The MEWS is even color-coded to facilitate its use. So, the message to the bedside nurses is *"We do not think you have the intellect and competence to identify patients who need critical attention but that's alright; just follow the yellow brick road... ...and, when it turns pink, call the RRT!"* They should

	SCORE	MET CALL	3	2	1	0	1	2	3	MET CALL
	ZONE	PINK	ORANGE	GOLD	YELLOW	WHITE	YELLOW	GOLD	ORANGE	PINK
PARAMETER	Respiratory Rate	<5	5-8			9-20		21-30	31-35	>35
	Systolic Blood Pressure	<70	70-79	80-89	90-99	100-180		>180		
	Heart Rate	<40	40-49			50-100	101-110	111-130	131-140	>140
	4 Hour Urine Output		<80	80-120		>120				
	Level of Consciousness	Unresponsive	Pain	Agitation/ Confusion	Voice	Alert				

Figure 15-2
MEWS Scale at Wellington Hospital. New Zealand

have added that, in between RRT calls, nurses should continue to fill out useless forms that no one reads. Ha! And this is from the group most vocal about being treated like professionals.

The decisive delivery of definitive care requires a physician; nothing else will do! The best approach, in my opinion, is that of the original intent: To expand the responsibilities of the cardiac arrest (i.e. code) team. This guarantees, in any hospital, that one of the physicians who is available 24/7 has the opportunity to deliver definitive care on a moments notice. Any other strategy that relies on non-physician personnel results in nothing other than delays in treatment.

Although I have covered two clearly downgrading policies and protocols, hospitals abound with numerous others that are less complex but more ubiquitous. One example is known as an "Oxygen Administration Protocol" and it allows nurses and respiratory therapists to administer different levels of oxygen depending on the patient's oxygenation measurements at the bedside. So, a patient whose oxygenation is declining will be progressively given greater amounts of supplemental oxygen until a limit is reached. The problem is that, while this is happening, no one is worrying about the cause for the need of oxygen, the underlying problem that eventually will need correction. This, of course will be a job for the RRT!

In summary, hospital policies and protocols represent the smaller sibling of the measures described in Chapter 14 at a national level. They symbolize the bread and butter of the administrators and middle nursing managers' jobs descriptors about meddling with clinical activities they do not clearly understand. The ICU open visitation policy, a failure from day one, has transformed the care environment into public markets, without control or situational awareness. The result is nurses being distracted from patient care, families inappropriately interacting with physicians and illegally being exposed to other patients' confidential information. The RRTs are a clear example of the uncritical thinking process that plagues the committee operations of the hospitals, the presumptuousness of the administrators, and the lack of prioritization of real quality indicators. The downgrading effect of both policies and protocols must not be underestimated, particularly since a solution may be quite possible.

16

Emergencies

"...Brought out the villagers three or four times by crying out, 'Wolf!' 'Wolf!' and when his neighbors came to help him, laughed at them for their pains. The Wolf however, did truly come at last. The Shepherd boy, now really alarmed, shouted in an agony of terror, but no one paid any heed to his cries, nor rendered assistance."

"The Shepherd Boy and the Wolf"
Aesop
Greek Writer
(620 – 564 BC)

I have carried a pager with me most of my adult life. Just like everyone who has done the same, long ago I came to grips with the reality that such device was part of my profession; that it was required for me to be available to attend individuals in acute distress, whether in the emergency department (ED) or in the intensive care unit (ICU). Most of us have seen this responsibility as part of the deal, part of the contract we have made with the patients we serve and, frankly, we have not given it another thought over the course of time. Originally, pagers were introduced in order to allow physicians to be reachable once they were not inside the hospital, where overhead paging was the main form of alert. It was implicitly understood that the use of the pagers to summon physicians meant that the reasons for their use were of significant importance to warrant such an interruption upon the life of medical professionals.

As time has gone by, however, the practice of "paging" has snowballed into a matter of convenience to be able to get in touch with the physician no matter what the reason for doing so is. This transformation and *downgrading* of the concept of an emergency has come to the point that it is difficult to distinguish when one is needed versus when one is just wanted. As we have seen in other chapters of this book, the progressive dilution of education, expertise and competence serves as the infrastructure for behavioral changes that include the inability to differentiate a true emergency from simply a nuisance question, and appropriately act according to which one is operating. The infractions that we witness on a daily basis to the unwritten understanding that emergency calls need to be so, represent the product of equations with multiple variables that must be individually addressed, particularly education, leadership and entitlements. In the next few pages, I will discuss the different aspects of this problem, and the various reasons why at present, paraphrasing my old mentor, life is nothing but *"a series of random intrusions on planned effort"*.

An emergency, by definition, is a clinical situation that demands immediate attention, particularly because if not addressed, unnecessary harm may come to the patient. It is a plea for the physician to hastily pivot, and shift the priorities of his attention in order to change the course of a clinical scenario that unravels in a downhill direction. However, it is not a query that is posed to a physician for the convenience of the patient, his family, or any other member of the clinical team. This working definition is the one that all of us accepted when we entered the practice of medicine, as well as later when we were handed a pager to carry around 24/7. Therefore, it has been our expectation that when the piercing sound of the pager diverts our attention from whatever task we are involved at that moment, and which we are forced to drop expeditiously, the cause of such distraction is worthy of the effort and energy expenditure. Furthermore, the distraction should have a clearer urgency and greater importance than the original task that it interrupted. However, a cursory review of the calls I receive in any one-week shows that approximately 70-80% are not true emergencies (i.e. *faux* emergencies), and could have been addressed in the context of a better priority scheme. Moreover, it is possible to identify various types of these *faux* emergencies, each with its own common and recognizable setting. Let's look at some of them (by no means is my list all-inclusive):

1) The Nursing Afterthought. This is one of the most irritating of the scenarios. It works like this: The physician makes clinical rounds and addresses all issues, writes all the orders, and leaves the nursing unit to go see patients elsewhere. Within a matter of minutes (usually less than 15!) he is paged back to answer a query that the nurse failed to raise during rounds. There are two variants of this: One in which the nurse was simply nowhere to be found during rounds and arrived after the physician had left, and the other in which the nurse simply forgot to bring up the issue in question despite the fact that he was present. In the former, it is even more

irritating that no communications took place to cover the absent nurse during clinical rounds.

2) The "Education" Afterthought. This *faux* emergency is similar to the previous but is due to the fact that either the patient or his family decided to ask one more question after the physician had left the nursing unit. Yes, I know, they are within their right to do so. However, my criticism has to do with their sense of entitlement that a physician has to be available for them no matter how many times they want him to be so. Also, their need for instant gratification, regardless of whomever else's care they may be interrupting. Finally, their unwillingness to write down questions and have them ready for the next physician's visit. This scenario is usually compounded by the nurses' failure to properly advise the patient and the family about the most reasonable approach to their query, as well as the recent transformation of hospitals' cultures from a service to a hospitality model (i.e. Medicine *à la Carte*).

3) The Entitled Family Member. This scenario is most common in the context of large families that include individuals unwilling to discuss the patient's status with him or with other family members who have been previously briefed by the physician. These family members typically appear on the scene after rounds are concluded and the physician has moved on to other nursing units; ordinarily demanding to speak with the physician directly and immediately. In my experience, the worst offenders are family members who preface their demands with statement such as *"I am a nurse!"* Really? By now the reader should easily predict how immensely

unimpressed I am by such an unsolicited confession. My criticism of this scenario centers on the fact that the information these latecomers seek has already been made available. They are just too self-centered to learn it from other family members and insist on being the center of attention. They absolutely *must understand* the patient's situation; they are more qualified than anyone else in the family to interpret the information; they have a point of view that goes along with their egos. This narcissistic approach to clinical communication, indicative of underlying character flaws, is typically accompanied by a low threshold to initiate a complain campaign against the physician if their wishes are not granted *ipso facto*.

4) The Therapeutic Pharmacist. This scenario is also one that most commonly follows clinical rounds. The physician has left the nursing unit after writing all orders, only to be paged within 20 minutes or so because, upon sending a certain order to the pharmacy, the receiving pharmacist has decided to practice medicine without a license. The typical conversation includes some statement such as *"Pharmacy refuses to fill the antibiotic because the patient is allergic to a similar class of antibiotics!"* At this point, after the desire to strangle the pharmacist subsides, the physician is forced to point out that the so-called allergy is simply a drug administration discomfort, and that this information was made available during rounds. One more unnecessary *faux* emergency call; one more unnecessary treatment delay! My criticism of this scenario is based upon the overreaching pharmacists insist on having, without assuming the ultimate responsibility for the care of the patient, and

which I have addressed elsewhere in the book (see Chapter 10).

5) The Urgent Comfort. This scenario stems directly from a combination of patient entitlement and the cultural changes that have transformed hospitals into pseudo-hotels. Typically, the physician is paged at any time of the day or night because the patient wants a laxative, or a sedative, or simply a medication his neighbor suggested he should be given. I can assure you, at 2:00 A.M., this type of call is anything but welcome. Unfortunately, satisfying the every whim of the patient has a direct impact on patient satisfaction scores, an important metric in today's proposed quality of care environment. After all, even the federal government has introduced this as one of their more recent indicators (see Chapter 14).

6) The Situational Unawareness. This one is directly related to nurses' lack of consideration and professionalism, at least in my opinion. Most physicians make rounds at predictable times on a daily basis. Therefore, queries that are not emergent, can be collected and raised during clinical rounds. Thus, I find it incredibly impervious to have the physician paged 30-60 minutes before he physically arrives in the nursing unit to make rounds, just to ask whether the patient can get out of bed or not, or some other question whose answer is not critically needed at that very moment.

The implications of *faux* emergency calls are multiple and carry fairly negative connotations. The most obvious is illustrated by the quote at the beginning of the chapter. Misusing a mechanism designed to summon the attention of physicians due to real medical emergencies and expanding it to include calls triggered by non-emergent circumstances eventually leads to dulling of the senses in response to unexpected hospital calls. Therefore, sooner or later the physician finds himself in the unfamiliar circumstance of not giving unexpected calls the priority the may require, simply out of the habit of receiving what amounts to mounds of nuisance calls.

The second implication is the waste of time and energy, as well as their diversion away from another activity pertinent to another patient, possibly one of a higher clinical priority. These *faux* emergency calls are definite interruptions, a fact that does not seem to be well appreciated. It is not as if physicians are sitting around doing nothing, just waiting to be paged! On the contrary, at the rate the present system is going, physicians are predictably seeing patients at almost any time day or night. To call a physician, without taking into consideration of the interruption caused in someone else's medical care, is thoughtless and conceited.

So, why does this problem exist? What are the factors that have led to the transformation of the strategies for handling emergencies? I submit that the current state of affairs is simply part of cultural changes induced by regulatory changes and educational reforms. As I have argued before, the dumbing down process to which we have subjected nurses cannot result in anything but their lack of competence at the bedside. This translates into difficulties recognizing true from *faux* emergencies; what needs to be handled immediately from what does not; when to call the physician and when to wait. This inability to critically assess clinical priorities is compounded by two other factors: The time we force them to spend fulfilling regulator mandates by completing forms and collecting meaningless data, and the availability of alternative professionals to whom they can "pass the buck" (Figure 12-1). All of these factors converge to create a conditioning on the nurses by which they react out of fear and insecurity. In fact, the mere term given to abnormal laboratory results (i.e. *"Panic Values"*) underscores the behavior resulting from receiving these results on the nursing unit. Not uncommonly, this leads to the juvenile practice of paging a physician and entering "911" in the pager, to indicate, *"I really, really mean for this to be an emergency call!"* But, does this make sense? Not if you think about it! In fact, it is the opposite of sensible! One of the characteristics of any professional is that of maintaining composure in the face of a crisis. In the past, when teaching students and residents how to handle emergencies, the traditional lesson was: *"The first thing you do is take your own pulse!"* Unless you are able to keep yourself cool, calm and collected, you will be of no use to the patient in trouble. If instead we teach nurses the occurrence of "panic" situations, and fail to provide them with the knowledge and skills to handle them, we should not be surprised that they call physicians indiscriminately at all times and for all reasons.

However, the most egregious manifestation of the cultural changes that negatively impact how emergencies are handled relates to the misguided practice of hospitals of managing emergency schedules as if they belonged in a clinic (Figure 16-1). No, I am not kidding! At a time when there is still a national crisis due to the overcrowding of EDs; when government regulators have used the overutilization of EDs by the "uninsured" as one of the rationalizations to pass more controlling legislation such as the Affordable Care Act (ACA) (i.e. Obamacare), their argument being that by going to the ED their care would be much more expensive. However, the metamorphosis of our system into a hospitality industry, catering to every whim of patients, has gotten us to the point illustrated n Figure 16-1. Patients can now go to a website and request a "reservation" in the ED so they can be seen with minimal delay; they can essentially "schedule" their emergencies so they are not an inconvenience; they get a service not unlike the one I get in www.OpenTable.com when I want to secure a table in my favorite restaurant. As you can see, there are even billboards by the highway that "invite"

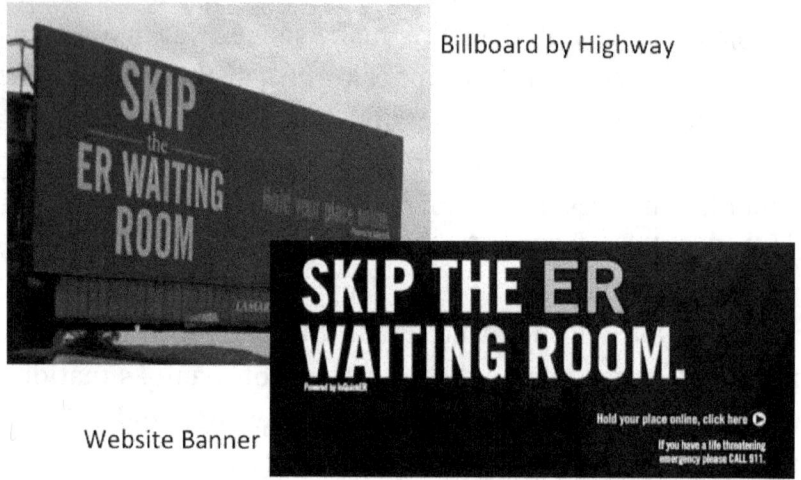

Figure 16-1
Invitation to Come to the ER by Appointment

people to use the system. In fact, some of these billboards have giant clocks that indicate the waiting time in the ED! So, the next time someone complains about the overcrowding of EDs, remember that the hospitals are not necessarily the victims but are part of the problem.

In summary, there is currently a profoundly distorted view of how to prioritize medical emergencies, both from the perspective of bedside nursing as well as from that of the arbiters of hospital culture: The administrators! In general, the transformation of hospital work from a philosophy of patient care to that of clinical serfdom provides the underpinnings of behavioral changes that are shortsighted, not prioritized, and in my view downright unprofessional. Although the bedside nurses constitute the group with the largest volume of violations to time honored, unwritten rules regarding the summoning of physicians for alleged clinical emergencies, the truth is that their comportment is nothing but the expected consequence of the cultural and regulatory changes imposed on them from the higher echelons. If we cannot clearly differentiate true from *faux* emergencies, can we really prioritize the delivery of care?

17

Pain

"Pain and death are a part of life. To reject them is to reject life itself."

Havelock Ellis
British Physician and Psychologist
(1859 - 1939)

An old professor of mine used to say, *"The only people without back pain are people who have no backs!"* At the time, I was too young and inexperienced to fully appreciate the wisdom of such a statement. Over the years, however, it has become clear that the subject of pain is the focus of the lives of countless human beings. As such, I found this to be one of the most difficult chapters to write as I was working in this book. On one hand, I do not want the reader to think that I am completely heartless, devoid of compassion, or that I do not have any empathy for suffering patients. On the other hand, the development of a subculture revolving around pain needs to be exposed and discussed openly, pointing out the factors that have motivated such an evolution, and the unintended consequences of the decisions that have been made along the way.

I will begin our discussion with the premise in the caption at the beginning of the chapter. Pain *is* a part of life! There can be no life without pain being present at one point or another. So how is it that such a common phenomenon has become the center of attention of millions of people, and has evolved to the point of having created an entire medical field around it? An entire medical field! Think about it! Most medical specialties exist in the context of illnesses common to a specific organ system (e.g. gastroenterology, urology) or a specific service (e.g. anesthesiology, emergency medicine). There's only one medical specialty whose existence revolves around a single symptom: *Pain Management!* In my opinion, the only way we can explain how a single symptom led to the creation of a field of medicine, one that continues to flourish at the time of this writing, implicates uncritical medical thinking, the public's sense of entitlement, a lack of clinical perspective, and politics, tons and tons of politics! Therefore, as we plow through a topic such as this, where emotions run high and contaminate many an intellectual discussion, it is best if we dissect it slowly and identify its parts prior to taking a critical look at the present status in the context of these determining facets.

To begin, as we noted earlier, pain is a symptom (i.e. something only the patient feels). It is an alarm system by which the body signals that something is wrong. Something that must be attended to, corrected, and its effects reversed in order for the alarm (i.e. the pain) to be silenced. Therefore, all treatment of pain must be undertaken in the context of this model. Otherwise, all we are doing is covering the source of the problem and we run the risk of making matters worse. It is only after the underlying cause of the pain has been reasonably identified, that we can fairly assess the realistic context of the symptom and how to prioritize its management. Let's face it; we have the pharmacologic means to get rid of nearly any amount of pain. So the issue is not whether we can do it but rather, what is the proportional and reasonable therapeutic response in each clinical circumstance. In other words, is it really necessary to use a shotgun to kill a fly? Just because we have access to powerful narcotics does not mean we should use them indiscriminately. This, of course, is not the most popular opinion within the current pain management culture. Here lies the clinical struggle we will expose in the following pages, together with the healthcare downgrading effects of current trends (remember our discussion in Chapter 6 about the use of narcotics in the context of polypharmacy).

A second issue we must point out in the context of choosing the therapeutic approach to pain is whether the strategy carries the risk of endangering the patient's well being (directly or indirectly)? Medicine, just like Economics, is a perfect field for the application of the proverbial *"There ain't no such thing as a free lunch!"* (TANSTAAFL). Every step we take, every decision we make, every strategy we choose, carries with it a set of consequences, both intended and unintended. Some of these are deleterious and may overwhelm any positive effect of our actions. Pain management is ideally suited to illustrate this type of interaction, as we will discuss in the following pages. Suffice it to say that, even in the best of circumstances, the most reasonable of decisions can lead to unexpected and sometimes unforeseen outcomes. Having said this, it is time for yet another anecdote as a form of illustration.

Circa 1983, as I was staffing the neurology clinic at the Veterans Administration (VA) hospital in St. Louis, I received a phone call to inform me that my father (who at the time of this writing has been deceased for almost 10 years) had to be taken to a local emergency room in Florida with acute abdominal pain suggestive of appendicitis. The emergency physician had made the correct presumptive diagnosis and promptly administered an opioid analgesic to relieve my father's discomfort while arranging for a surgeon to see him. Unfortunately, the patient being how he was, decided that since he no longer had pain, he was ready to go home. Predictably, this led to a conflict that resulted in my father signing himself out of the emergency room against medical advice (AMA). The consequences of such an action were also quite predictable: As the effect of the analgesic subsided, his abdominal pain returned with a vengeance. Only that, by then, so much time had elapsed that his appendix had ruptured, causing peritonitis (i.e. widespread abdominal infection) and rapidly endangering his life. To compound the problem, the emergency room staff that had seen him earlier that day now wanted to have nothing to do with him, in my opinion rightfully so. Thus, from 1200 miles away, I found myself in the necessity to make several phone calls and call in some favors to get him the care he needed. Although the ultimate outcome of this misadventure was good, it should be illustrative of the problem we are about to address in the following pages: the treatment of pain, without taking into consideration the overall requirements of the patient, represents incomplete, naïve, and suboptimal medical management! To be clear, I do not think the physician in my anecdote did anything wrong. On the contrary, I agree that patients need not suffer pain unnecessarily in circumstances such as this. In this case, the problem had to do with the patient's expectations and personal perspective regarding his medical issues.

Back to our discussion, to choose the treatment of pain as the primary goal of management, rather than the correction of its cause is, in principle, neither a logical nor a sound practice. If we accept this assertion as true, then we must examine the current status of pain management in our country in its light. Doing so will rapidly lead us to conclude that we have derailed this aspect of medical care in order to satisfy wrongful expectations and gullible pseudo-intellectual arguments, while foolishly ignoring the potentially damaging consequences (intended and unintended) of the indiscriminate utilization of powerful analgesics. At this point, it is important for the reader to realize the relationship between the topic in this chapter and those that address problem-oriented medical diagnosis (POMD) (Chapter 3), polypharmacy (Chapter 6), entitlements (Chapter 18), and medication side effects (Chapter 20). In fact, this is a vastly reaching subject that insinuates itself into nearly every aspect of medical practice. We must even point out its bearing on medical malpractice (Chapter 9) since we know of at least one case in which a physician was successfully sued because of failure to provide sufficient analgesia and therefore causing "unnecessary pain and suffering".

The relationship of pain to POMD is fairly evident; after all, it is easy to use "pain" as an entry in the problem list of any patient. Typically, it is not used in its generic form but rather attached to more specific issues, for example "chronic low back pain" or simply "chronic pain". The reader should quickly notice, as I pointed out in Chapter 3, that those types of entries are noncommittal and fraught with problems relative to their evaluation and management. To leave pain as a freestanding equivalent to any diagnosis is to lose sight of the importance of tailoring treatment to the underlying condition that causes any symptom. It opens a path of least resistance, which in this case ends up with the chronic prescription of powerful narcotics in an attempt to alleviate a painful condition that could have been completely annulled by treating its cause. Just as I have mentioned elsewhere, the intellectual laziness that underscores such an approach is widespread, and its downgrading result on the practice of medicine continues to grow exponentially.

As we continue to explore the effect of considering pain as an independent target for treatment, we cannot but stumble into the protean consequences of polypharmacy. We are at a point now where patients treated for pain, irrespective of its cause, concurrently received medications believed to exert a complementary effect, with very little regard to the fact that their side effects will also complement each other. As such, it is not uncommon in my practice to see patients who have difficulties with arousal, attention, memory, orientation, and even motor performance as a result of the effect of multiple pain medications given concomitantly. In fact, one of the most common reasons for requesting neurologic consultation in hospitalized patients is the infamous *"altered mental status".* This wastebasket term, good for nothing since it is typically among the top positions within yet another uncritical problem list, in my experience is 90% of the time the result of polypharmacy designed to alleviate pain, anxiety or both. This is particularly true in the elderly and the very young.

The culture of pain management is such that it has resulted in a variety of very illogical practices. First and foremost is the obsession with quantifying pain. As we noted earlier, a symptom is something only the patient can feel. Therefore, any attempt at creating an objective measure of it from the perspective of an observer is simply ludicrous. That has not stopped the *intelligentsia* from generating a variety of pain "scales" (Figure 17–1). The illustration depicts the two most important type of scales presently used across the land. The one on top is known as the Wong-Baker FACES Scale, and was introduced by a pediatric nurse for the purpose of assessing pain in children who were too young to describe the intensity of their discomfort. It is a perfect example of how a reasonably good idea can be perverted to such degree that its ubiquitous presence in all medical charts is nothing but the logotype of uncritical thinking. The stupidest of them

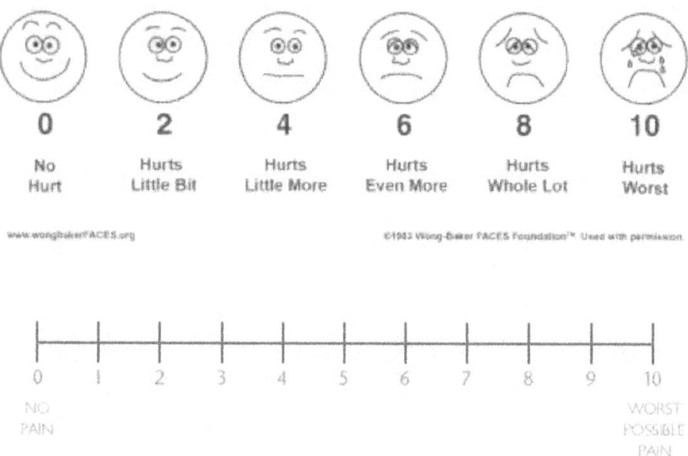

Figure 17-1
The Most Commonly Used Pain Scales

all, however, is the one on the bottom of figure 17–1, which endeavors to assign a score to the degrees of pain. Its absurdity is so evident that makes you wonder how is it that it has become the most widely used in daily practice. Think about it; assigning a numerical value to something that is impossible to quantify just so we can feel good about ourselves, can "relate" to the discomfort of the patient, and have an idea how much analgesics to administer. The assumption in which the use of pain scales is based defies logic and common sense: *A pain score has the same meaning in all patients!* Let me place this idiotic premise into context. By definition, "quantity" is the property that confers an order of magnitude that allows objective comparison. By inference, "quantification" is the act of assessing, measuring or determining such a property under specific circumstances. For example, determining the height of an individual to be 5' 7" is an objective act that results in a measurement that is identical for every individual of the same height. However, this is not the case when it comes to pain scales since no measurement is taking place. The score is simply the patient's "perception" of the degree of pain, which derives from a subjective assessment.

Despite the undisputable rationality of my argument, however, the assessment of pain has gained significant notoriety over the last few years, to the point that the California Legislature has introduced a bill (AB 791) that compels medical schools to include pain management in their curriculum as a requirement to seek a medical license in that state. Moreover, it requires organizations to include the assessment of pain as a *"fifth vital sign"* (following the ones traditionally recorded: heart rate, temperature, respiratory rate, and blood pressure). But wait! I thought that *signs* were those findings obtained objectively by physical examination. So, how is it that a subjective item can be included in this list? Ah! There is a story behind this! In 1996, in his presidential address to the American Pain Society (APS), James Campbell, M.D. made the following statement: *"...vital signs are taken seriously... ... if pain where assessed with the same zeal as all other vital signs are, it would have a much better chance of being treated properly."* This is all that was needed! A comment regarding how attentive people should be to the assessment of pain was the catalyst of a firestorm destined to end in additional regulatory controls. Shocking! By 1998, the Veterans Administration (VA) began a national strategy to improve pain management entitled "Pain as the 5th Vital Sign", and centered it around the use of numeric rating scales for pain. Following this, our old friend the Joint Commission (TJC) introduced pain management standards for their accredited facilities in 2001. Even more recently, another one of the usual suspects, the Institute of Medicine (IOM) published a report described as *"A Blueprint for Transforming Prevention, Care, Education, and Research"* (note the unswerving reference to "transformation"). The rest is history! At present, nurses get browbeaten if they do not insist repeatedly that patients tell them what their pain score is. In fact, it is no longer acceptable to expect the patient to volunteer that he has pain (a reasonable expectation on the part of any of us who has ever suffered pain). No; open-ended questions such as *"how are you feeling?"* are being replaced by leading questions such as *"how much pain do you have?"* This is as much of a leading question as the often quoted *"Do you enjoy beating your wife?"* One with implicit expectations and assumptions. There seems to be a lack of understanding that a conversation with a patient is part of how we examine them, and that volunteering of certain information provides additional important knowledge regarding their medical and psychological status. Ironically, the inclusion of pain assessment as a "5th vital sign" has been shown to have no beneficial effect on the treatment of pain, at least in VA hospitals. Thus, this is yet another example of government surrogates increasing the energy expenditure at the bedside without improving the outcome of the patients. It reminds me of the proverbial *"peeing in a dark pair of pants"* (i.e. it gives you a warm feeling, but no one can tell the difference!).

As we continue our discussion, I want to take a moment to expand on the physical and psychological aspects of pain perception. As a working definition, *pain is an unpleasant sensory and emotional experience associated with actual or potential tissue damage*. Pain is somewhat different from other forms of perception (e.g. vision, hearing) in that it includes a rather urgent and primitive quality with strong affective and emotional aspects. Furthermore, *its intensity is affected by a variety of factors in such a way that the same stimulus may result in different responses, in different individuals, even under similar circumstances*. There goes the whole concept of pain scales! Now, back to our fundamental discussion, the starting point of pain perception begins with the existence of specialized organ receptors called nociceptors (from Latin *nocere* 'to harm' + RECEPTOR). Interestingly, the stimulation of these receptors does not necessarily lead to the perception of pain. In fact, the latter is a product of how the brain processes, abstracts, and elaborates the input from the nociceptors. Clear example of this is seen in battle, where soldiers often do not feel pain until they have been safely removed from danger. In any case, the activation of nociceptors produces electrical impulses that are transmitted via the peripheral nerves to the spinal cord, within which they ascend to the brain to be processed. There is significant evidence at the present time that the parts of the brain that are involved in the processing of pain are not only those within the sensory system itself but also others that are part of the *limbic system*. The latter encompasses a group of structures with a major role in emotional experiences. And so, we see that the phenomenon of pain perception includes a significant emotional component responsible for the variability of the effect of the same stimulus among the patient population. I see this everyday in my practice! In order to perform cerebral catheterizations, we most commonly access the brain blood vessels through the femoral artery (i.e. the artery in the groin area). It is fascinating how the same operator, using the same exact needle, and performing the same exact injection of local anesthetic, elicits so different a response from each patient; all the way from almost jumping off the table, to not showing any reaction at all! I cannot overemphasize the emotional component of pain perception because it is closely tied to the expectations of the patient for his medical care, particularly in the long-term.

And this brings us to the center of our controversy: *Chronic Pain*! Although nearly everybody seems to be in agreement as to what *Acute Pain* represents, chronic pain is a complex subject, fraught with misunderstandings, passionate arguments, blind advocacy, and political rhetoric. Whereas acute pain typically results from an easily recognizable injury to tissue (just as the example of my father I described above), chronic pain often times has a much more elusive substrate. A perfect example of this phenomenon is *Fibromyalgia*, a highly popularized diagnosis for which there is little if any evidence of its existence as an entity separate from depression. I am sure some of the readers will disagree with my statement, but I can assure you that after reviewing the so-called "science" behind this diagnosis, I am completely convinced that it is part of the psychopathology I described in Chapter 6. But enough of this; it is not my intention to turn this chapter into a fibromyalgia debate.

At present, the working definition of chronic pain is that which *"persists or occurs for more than three months"* according to the two most vocal organizations championing its cause: the International Association for the Study of Pain (IASP) and the European Federation of IASP Chapters (EFIC).

In principle, I do not disagree with such a concept and therefore I will use it to provide a framework for the rest of our discussion. The reader should quickly realize that we are using a relatively all-encompassing definition, predictably leading to the conclusion that what we call "chronic pain patients" represent a very heterogeneous group of people. As such, some of my criticisms regarding the current culture of chronic pain management do not apply to every single individual that suffers from chronic pain. For example, on one extreme, I am of the opinion that patients with certain diagnoses characteristically associated with severe and disabling pain (e.g. cancer, rheumatoid arthritis), and for which there is no cure or reversal, should not be denied the benefit of analgesics (even narcotics) in order to optimize their quality of life. However, notice that I did not say the complete relief of pain. The reason is simple; it may or may not be possible to achieve this goal! Moreover, the price to pay for complete pain relief in terms of treatment side effects may be unacceptable. It is precisely for this reason that the patient–physician relationship in these cases needs to be close but also clear in terms of goals of treatment. As I said earlier, to expect one to live completely and constantly free of pain is unrealistic. That said, the comfort of the patient in order to optimize his quality of life is not only a reasonable goal but also a measure of quality of care.

The problem I have stems from a statement made by EPIC in 2001: *"Pain is a major healthcare problem… …chronic and recurrent pain is a specific healthcare problem, a disease in its own right"*. Those of us who have studied neurophysiology will have to drink gallons of Kool-Aid® in order to believe such rhetoric. I challenge such an assertion and submit that chronic pain is also a symptom of something that is wrong physically, psychologically, or both. Physical disorders that cause chronic pain may not have a cure, or a form of reversal as we noted earlier. It is in these cases where I have absolutely no quarrel with effective chronic pain management by someone who has the expertise to tailor the treatment to the individual patient. In these cases, I also do not disagree with the strategic utilization of narcotics if necessary. However, patients whose pain either has no recognizable physical substrate, or whose pain is clearly out of proportion to the alleged injury, in my view belong within the realm of psychiatry since almost invariably they have concurrent or underlying emotional disorders. I actually think that we do these patients a disservice by not clearly and openly discussing this very fact with them. There is a stigma associated with the idea that *"it's all in your head"* and this is a statement I have never made to a patient from my practice. It is unnecessary, inaccurate, and disrespectful. That said, the implication that such a stigma extends to the lack of need for psychiatric or psychological intervention is also unfair, and the failure to introduce these aspects of treatment to the patient's management program is just as bad as withholding narcotics from a patient with cancer pain. After being in medical practice for over three decades, I have come to the conclusion that the secret to a healthy life is *happiness!* Happy people seem to withstand illness much better and with the least negative impact; conversely, we do not seem to be able to make unhappy people get better regardless of how hard we try! This distinction could not be clearer than in the chronic pain population. The emotional and psychological components of their condition are real, and they help create a vicious cycle that perpetuates their misery and interferes with their improvement, narcotics or not! It is not a coincidence that the pain in these patients responds to the use of antidepressant medications, or that many of the medications currently advertised as indicated for chronic pain are also useful in the treatment of depression.

Now, a word about the magnitude of the problem and the downgrading effect of the government surrogates' interventions; once again we see the hand of the IOM in publicizing the "crisis" that needs regulatory meddling and transformation. The IOM report lists certain facts as the justification for the changes recommended, including that at least 116 million adults in our country are burdened by chronic pain. Also, estimates of approximately $500-600 billions in national economic cost associated with this condition. Interestingly, they recognize the problem of the widespread abuse of opiates but they also embrace the IASP/EFIC opinion that chronic pain is a disease in itself. I think these two positions are very difficult to reconcile and to forcefully do so is a recipe for disaster. If you think I am exaggerating consider the following statistics:

- As of 2010, approximately 7.0 million persons (2.7% of the population) were abusing psychotherapeutic drugs, primarily pain medications (5.1million).

- Among adolescents, prescription medications are the most commonly abused illicit drugs, particularly opiates.

As we covered in Chapter 6, the problem of the widespread utilization of medications that alter neurologic function, whether indicated or not, is aggravated by the transformation of the system into one of avoiding an honest and clear discussion about the psychological component of chronic pain, and the need to look beyond pharmacologic interventions in order to provide a reasonable management strategy for these patients.

In summary, at the present time in our country there is a palpable cultural clash relative to the management of pain. There is the perception that patients must be treated to the point where they experience absolutely no pain, almost irrespective of the consequences, without considering the fact that the most important aspect of the treatment of pain is to address its underlying cause. Although it is possible to find suggestions about this latter point in the context of managing acute pain, the same subject is not so clearly addressed with respect to chronic pain. The heterogeneity of the patient population suffering from chronic pain is also not well defined when certain comments and recommendations are being made. Although certainly there is no excuse for not maximizing pain control, particularly in patients with a terminal illness or an incurable condition, such a goal should not be confused with the indiscriminate utilization of treatment strategies whose side effects overwhelm any potential benefit. The idea that chronic pain is a disease in itself is misguided and fails to take into account psychological causative factors that require specialized treatment. Furthermore, it results in an imperfect, incomplete, and dishonest approach to these patients, leading to unnecessary and excessive use of narcotics with its damaging consequences. Unless we take a hard look at the fact that the most important aspect of the care of the chronic patient rests in his relationship with his physician, and do away with gimmicks such as pain scales, our approach to these patients may be compliant with government regulations, but it will also be useless.

CULTURAL AND REGULATORY DOWNGRADING

18

Entitlements

"We the unwilling, led by the unknowing, are doing the impossible for the ungrateful. We have done so much, for so long, with so little, that we are now qualified to do anything with nothing"

Mother Teresa of Calcutta
Albanian-born Indian Missionary and Nobel Laureate
(1910 - 1997)

We live in a society riddled with entitlements. Don't believe me? Just think about the fact that, at the time of this writing, approximately 50% of the United States population does not pay taxes and yet, they are entitled to benefit from the same America that those of us who pay taxes get. Moreover, to add insult to injury, the present administration claims that we are still not paying our "fair share", and they are fixated in siphoning more of our income to continue to fund government growth and failed social programs. The predictable result of this political and economic philosophy is that we are cultivating generations of individuals whose life as they see it is "owed to them" by the rest of us. Do you think these people view healthcare differently? Dream on!

I certainly was not present at the time of their meeting but I am fairly confident that the founding fathers did not intend for our society to follow this path. So, even though you may think I am digressing, there is a point to this short soapbox. Healthcare is not an exception when it comes to the negative effects of an entitlement culture and, as we will discuss in the next few pages, the implications for healthcare entitlement are financial, social and political, all having a negative impact on patient care. How did we get to this point? Until 1965, medical care in our country did not require the involvement of the government. There were hospitals in all communities across the land, provided by churches, temples, and other religious institutions; in addition, many counties and cities erected hospitals to provide care for the poor. I had the opportunity to witness the tail end of this cultural trend firsthand when I came to this country; in the early 1980's I worked in both the St. Louis City and the St. Louis County Hospitals. Thus, prior to the 1965 intrusion of Congress in healthcare as part of *The Great Society*, individuals were expected to provide it for themselves in the same manner as they were expected to provide everything else since the foundation of the country. However, by virtue of creating Medicare and Medicaid, Congress began a process of progressive intervention and control of the type of care patients get, and its price. Such a process continued with the Health Maintenance Organization (HMO) Act of 1973, and includes Congress' latest accomplishment: The Affordable Care Act (ACA) (i.e. Obamacare). And so, unless something dramatic changes after the upcoming November election, the ACA promises to confer the government the power to regulate nearly all affairs relative to medical care in our country. In and of itself this is an alarming thought, since it represents one of the most powerful forms of control a government can exert over the citizens of any country. These post-1965 interventions also led to the development of an entitlement mentality that pervades many aspects of our *downgraded* system. As we stated at the beginning of the chapter, although there are millions of people that earn their keep every day, there are almost just as many who think they are entitled to receive healthcare at someone else's expense. And that's just the beginning of this aspect of the problem...

The financial repercussions of the sense of entitlement displayed by patients and their families stem from some of the concepts I introduced in Chapter 1 and covered further in Chapter 7. The fact that, in the majority of instances, patients are responsible for only a small portion of the financial burden of the care they receive results in their lack of understanding of the true value (or even the perceived value) of the healthcare transactions involving them. This means that the patients' views of the direct cost of healthcare are tainted and not even in the same ballpark as reality. Thus, they demand, and demand, and demand some more, without giving a second thought to the actual cost of what they want to receive. Don't believe me? Well, try this: The next time you have to speak with your attorney over the phone in order to have him answer a legal question for you, ask him if he is answering your query for free. Chances are that he will promptly inform you that you will be receiving a bill for such a call in the near future. On the other hand, patients do not think twice about calling a physician's office without anticipating to be charged for the time spent on the phone. This happens even after hours, when the physician on call is expected to take calls from patients without compensation. Is this entitled behavior? I say it is unparalleled!

Well, perhaps not. The most egregious of the financial entitlements I have witnessed is that of the Medicaid patients and their behavior relative to their co-pay. The latter amounts to $1 (yes, one dollar) and, by law, it should be collected during each visit. Otherwise, the visit may be disallowed and the physician will never collect the additional $59 paid by Medicaid. Believe you me when I tell you that collecting that one-dollar is generally a big production. Typically, the exchange begins by the patient presenting himself at the clinic check-in station and explaining that he does not have the $1 co-pay. Curiously, this occurs while his $200 iPhone rings incessantly and as he stands in his brand new $200 Nike™ shoes. Upon being told that, by law, it is impossible for him to be seen without collecting the $1 co-pay, he commonly darts out the door to his Mercedes-Benz or Cadillac (I wish I were kidding!) only to return a few minutes later with the money. He then proceeds to toss the money across the counter, either in coins or as a half-torn $1 bill, with visible contempt. Next, to add insult to injury, he steps outside to smoke as part of his $10 (two-pack) per day habit. Mind you that I am referring to Alabama prices since, if he were to live in New York, the same habit would cost him almost $24 per day. Now, do you think this is a behavior of entitlement? Wait, don't answer, there is more! Time for another anecdote!

Just today, in my clinic, I saw a Medicaid patient for the second time ever. She is a 32 year-old woman who used to be under the care of one of my former partners due to recurrent headaches. Upon his retirement, the patient was moved to my care. I saw her for the first time about one year ago. In reading her medical record, I noted an entry from my partner that explicitly indicated how this patient had discontinued on her own the preventive medication prescribed and, guess what? She was having headaches again! Since her last appointment, she had been making rounds, visiting various emergency rooms and urgent care facilities around town, searching for the omnipresent narcotic injection for her headaches. I impressed upon her that this behavior was counterproductive and her best course of action was to be restarted on a preventive strategy. Somehow, she seemed agreeable and I prescribed another preventive medication (she claimed the previous one did not agree with her) and gave her a follow up visit two weeks later, so we could discuss her progress. Today, almost one year later she returns, not having shown up for her scheduled appointment without so much as a courtesy phone call. She is not taking the medication I prescribed, and has been making the same around town visits to urgent care facilities as before. When I called her on her behavior, pointing out that we had covered this before, and that there was no way for us to help her unless she followed through with the plan, she suddenly seemed offended and tried to imply that I was out of line for talking to her that way. Mind you that, at the same time, she has been trying to get long-term disability benefits based on the diagnosis of... ...You guessed it: Migraine!

Imagine that! Young individuals in the prime of their life, seeking to be supported by society on the basis of one of the most common conditions on the face of the planet; and one certainly not disabling. I wish I could say that this example is an exception, or a rarity, but it is not. On the contrary, we come face to face with this type of behavior more frequently every day. There are thousands of people out there looking for an angle, whether directly through

Social Security disability determinations or workmen's compensation, in order to cash in on the weaknesses of the system. In all fairness, however, they could not accomplish such feat without some help. It begins with the politicians who have helped set up the overregulated and bureaucratic systems that provides the framework for this type of behavior; it is complemented by the attorneys that represent these patients knowing there is no real disability, and it is finalized by the physicians who declare them disabled.

However, the financial implications of the current entitlement mentality are only a symptom of a much bigger behavioral problem; one that is also palpable in our everyday interactions with patients and their families. At the core of this entire problem lies a self-centered attitude that manifests itself in the context of a need for instant gratification. You will remember our description of the behaviors we observed in the intensive care units (ICU) (Chapter 15), which by no means are an exception but a perfect example of the topic at hand. One of the commonest examples has to do with waiting for the physician. The truth is that no one wants to wait, and the majority of us do not like making others wait. However, there is a widespread failure to understand that the reason why a patient waits is... ... wait for it... ... *Other patients*! It is almost impossible to make people understand that, while they're waiting for us, we are not sitting around finishing crossword puzzles! Typically, we are attending to patients who have issues of a higher priority than those of the person waiting. Most of us would be delighted to be sure that every one of these needs fit a very neat and predictable schedule; one that would allow us to fulfill our mission according to a predetermined plan. Unfortunately, such an expectation is unrealistic, particularly when there are so many demands placed on us from so many patients. Ironically, the patients that do the most complaining often want to be sure that when their turn to be seen comes around, we spend sufficient time with them. This frequently leads to additional frictions since, after sitting in our waiting area for one or two hours, their visit with the physician only lasts a few minutes. At this time, the reader may think that this is a very unfair deal for the patient in question. However, I would ask your indulgence in allowing me to walk you through additional thoughts that may place the entire problem in perspective.

I submit that the apparent conflict in the interaction described is nothing more than the product of wrongful expectations based upon an entitlement mentality. As I said, there's nothing pleasant about waiting for a physician for one or two hours; I understand that, appreciate it and largely regret it. However, if you have had a stroke, or heart attack, or cancer, and a visit with your physician is necessary to improve your chances of living a longer, productive and fulfilling life, a time investment such as that does not seem too bad. Even if you wait one hour to see your primary physician for your routine yearly checkup, the same principles also seem applicable. Moreover, since these visits are typically scheduled, it should be easy to plan some type of activity (e.g. reading a book) to make good use of the waiting time. From this perspective, we get to the *leitmotif* of the entitlement problem: *Personal Convenience!*

As it turns out, nearly any medical interaction that results in an inconvenience is frowned upon. The most common example is how phone calls are handled. I have covered some aspects of this problem in Chapter 7, as well as at the beginning of the present chapter. Patients and families insist on making phone calls to ask questions about the care of the patient, and to have these answered immediately. Even when they are told that someone is going to get with them as quickly as possible, they call repeatedly because *"no one has called back!"* This happens on a daily basis and there are instances in which we have 3-4 messages about the same subject within a matter of a few hours. Mind you, that none of these represent medical emergencies since our policy is to unequivocally direct those patients to go to the emergency department (ED) for immediate care. Interestingly, upon telling these people that the answer cannot be provided over the phone but that we would be glad to see the patient that same afternoon in the clinic to discuss the issue, they frequently decline. Why? Because it is inconvenient to pack your bags and come to clinic to be seen! However, it is much more convenient to make phone call after phone call, and terrorize the clinic staff by including unpleasant expletives into the conversation. Furthermore, if you look carefully at our discussions in Chapters 15 and 16, you will clearly recognize the specter of inconvenience written all over the behaviors of these people.

Now, going back to the scenario of waiting in clinic to be seen for a protracted period of time, just so you can spend a few minutes with the physician, let me address the latter issue. Somehow, somewhere in our healthcare culture, there seems to be an unwritten rule that is believed by patients and that equates quality of care with a time spending delivering it. In other words, there is the widespread notion that more time is better time! This obtuse point of view, without any reasonable basis of logic or historical evidence, results frequent disappointments. Let me take this opportunity to dispel this myth by using an analogy. *If your house were on fire, would you rather have the problem handled by the fireman who can put out the fire in 2 minutes, or by the one who will take one hour?* Without too much analysis, it should be self-evident that the speed of the former fireman is likely to result in more of the house being saved. Believe it or not, this applies quite well to medical care. For example, those of us who perform neurologic interventional procedures adhere by a principle that states *"Time on the table equals complications!"* This tells us that we are there to perform a task, and that this task should be carried out without distractions and with as little time expenditure as it is necessary. Any unnecessary time spent with the patient on the table is more likely to translate into additional problems. Another aspect of this topic is the fact that patients do not realize how lucky they are that we don't have to spend too much time with them. Typically, this means that they are well or improving; that we do not need to address new issues, order additional tests, interpret additional information, or change treatment strategies, all of which take extra time.

Another interesting twist of the entitlement mentality pervasive in our country has to do with *"End of Life"* discussions. Even though I am not at all a proponent of any type of rationing, I also have a realistic view of all we can and cannot do on behalf of patients once the dying process has begun. Let's start this part of our discussion from the political point of view. It was not too long ago when former Alaskan Governor Sarah Palin was criticized for a commentary relative to the existence of *"Death Panels"* within the ACA. Proponents of this legislation vehemently denied that such group existed at all. Of course, if you ask around, none of them have really read the text of the ACA! As it turns out, Obamacare includes a panel of 15 unelected members known as the Independent Payment Advisory Board (IPAB), whose responsibilities will include decisions regarding what services or procedures will be covered. If you don't think the

IPAB is just the tip of the rationing iceberg, you have not been paying attention! As much as I would hate seeing the government making life and death decisions on behalf of patients, I think it is important that we take a hard look at how the state of affairs is at present. The truth is that we do see patients and families that are most reasonable when it comes to decisions about the end of someone's life. Commonly though, we have serious issues with families (typically very large and boisterous ones) that absolutely want *"everything done!"* In Chapter 19, I would make clearer how such a statement is devoid of any reasonable knowledge but, for the time being, then let me place it in perspective. The statement in question is usually made by members of the family of a patient such as this:

An 85-year-old man who has lived a productive and fruitful life, and who happens to have had hypertension and diabetes. One week earlier he fell down and broke his hip. He was admitted to the hospital and, since then, has had one after another complication to no-fault of anyone involved in his care. He currently has pneumonia involving both lungs, with consequent difficulty breathing, he has had a stress related secondary heart attack, and his kidneys are slowly failing. Despite all efforts he seems to be slipping away.

Surely, this patient can be placed on a ventilator; more aggressive therapy can be provided including stronger antibiotics, and even place him on temporary dialysis to overcome the kidney dysfunction. However, is this reasonable? In the absence of the patient having had a living will (and sometimes despite of it!) we are forced to deal with a family with enormously unrealistic expectations that cannot be appeased in a rational manner. Believe me when I tell you that this is not a rare occurrence, and in my view it represents a flagrant example of the widespread entitlement attitude.

Two different lines of thought are relevant to dealing with this behavior: a) The justification for intensive care, and b) The inevitability of death. After having spent the bulk of my professional career roaming around ICUs, I can attest to the fact that being a patient in one of these units can be one of the most undignified experiences for a human being. To be half conscious, half naked and semi-restrained in a hospital bed, connected to several machines by means of tubes and cables of various sizes for days or weeks doesn't even begin to describe how difficult for anyone is to endure such an experience. What makes it worthwhile? There's only one answer: *Hope!* The hope that the patient will improve by means of all of our treatments to the point of regaining his ability to carry out the rest of his life with sufficient quality as he would have wanted. That's it! No mystery. The more we erode at the concept of having reasonable hope for recovery, the less justifiable it is to maintain a patient indefinitely under the circumstances described. Most professionals I know that have worked in intensive care share in this line of thought, and are quick to recognize when the care being delivered to the patient is futile. The concept of *futility* in medicine is a very important one, and one that requires honest introspection into our capabilities. Unfortunately, the entitlement mentality interferes with the effectiveness of the physician's advice to families in the context of futile care. It replaces trust and respect with suspicion and arrogance, failing to take into account that it is the wishes of the patient that should supersede those of anyone else involved in the care.

In regards to the second line of thought, I would like to point out that everyone is going to die! No matter what! We begin to die the moment we are born and the result is inexorable. Therefore, in recognizing this, we also come to the conclusion that medicine is never intended to prevent death, but simply to delay it when it appears to be occurring in an untimely or premature manner. Interestingly enough, when you think about this notion in the context of the patients such as the one described above, there comes a point during their care in which every task relative to their care simply delays the inevitable.

Interestingly, the response of our healthcare system to the entitlement mentality has been one of acquiescence. Due to the unfortunate importance of patient satisfaction scores as a surrogate measure of quality (see Chapters 11, 14 and 15), the powers that be at various levels have promoted the entitlement attitude by catering to it in what I refer to as *medicine à la Carte*. At present, patients and families are coached and encouraged to demand certain treatments and to expect that everyone within the medical team will be at their beck and call on a moments notice. Imagine what this does to the patient–physician relationship. It takes it from an equal partnership to one of intended servitude, and examples of this pattern abound. If you ask a patient, as I often do, who is his primary physician, the answer you are more likely to get is phrased in the following manner: *"I use Dr. Jones!"* Really? Does this sound like an equal level partnership to you? Make no mistake, these changes in the relationship between physicians and patients run very deep, and explain why a patient who does not like his physician is inclined to *"fire"* him.

Finally, a word about *Second Opinions!* This is perhaps one of the most misunderstood concepts in clinical medicine, and one of the most commonly involved in the context of entitled behavior. The reality is that second opinions were created as the means for a physician to ask another physician for another opinion (i.e. a fresh pair of eyes) about a puzzling clinical situation. It was never intended as the means for patients to go around shopping for someone to tell them what they want to hear! Yes, it is the right of any patient to seek another point of view about his diagnosis or proposed treatment. That said, I think it is imperative that he understands the implications and consequences of such an action:

1) Going spontaneously to seek another opinion is a breach of trust. The moment a patient seeks another physician's advice about what he has already been told, he is effectively stating, *"I am not convinced you are right, and I want some else to give me an opinion!"* The uncertainty that engenders such behavior is unequivocal and immediately changes the patient-physician relationship (Figure 1-1). Thus, a patient who proceeds this way must be prepared for the consequential change in relationship that it will cause, akin to saying to your spouse *"I am not convinced you are giving me what I need, and I want to try someone else!"* Most patients do not give this a second thought.

2) Seeking another opinion may increase uncertainty. There are only two possible outcomes of a second opinion: *agreement* or *disagreement* with the first one. If the former takes place, then what? Does the patient return to the original physician and say, *"Never mind! You were right and I want to continue being your patient!"* (Akin to *"It's alright honey, after trying it with someone else, I have*

> *decided that you do give me what I need!"*)? And, if there is a disagreement, how does the patient know which of the two opinions if the correct? And, if he decides that the original physician made more sense, does he return back (Akin to *"Honey, I am back! I tried it with someone else and she was not as good as you!"*)?

My point is that we have taken a concept meant to provide patients with an expanded expertise and made it into an opinion shopping mechanism by which patients often go around in search for statements that fit their expectations. Mind you that I think it is perfectly within their rights to do so; God knows that many patients recognize suboptimal medical care and are wise in seeking better advice. However, just like anything else in medicine, there is always another side to the coin, and patients need to fully understand all the variables in this equation.

In summary, the entitlement mentality that currently runs rampant in our society makes no exception for healthcare. Patients and families commonly display a self-centered and egotistical behavior, made worse by the need for instant gratification. As such, they demand undivided attention while ignoring the rights of other patients to have similar services. Moreover, they fail to realize that, unless they change and learn the realities of the inevitability of death, and the limitations of medicine, they will be directly affected by rationing decisions made by bureaucratic panels created by the government.

19

Patient Education

"It ain't ignorance that causes so much trouble; it's folks knowing so much that ain't so!"

Josh Billings
American Humorist and Lecturer
(1818 - 1885)

Do we want informed patients? Definitely! Is it our responsibility to teach them pharmacology? Molecular biology? Neuropathology? Absolutely not! And this is the dilemma we face on a daily basis; what is the boundary between providing patients with information that is important and relevant for them to have, and confusing matters by discussing concepts they are incapable of fully understanding? Once again, I do not have any quarrel with the fundamental idea of communicating information to patients. Frankly, an informed patient is more capable of assuming an active role in his care. However, just like many other good ideas I have discussed throughout the book, we have also gone too far in executing a strategy that covers this issue. In this context, we again find that the ubiquitous

Institute of Medicine (IOM) has called attention to yet another "crisis" in what they have chosen to name "Health Literacy". This is defined as *"the degree to which individuals have the capacity to obtain, process, and understand basic health information and services needed to make appropriate health decisions"*. I think it is important that we keep in mind this definition while we discuss this topic further in the following pages, because it will help understand the point that I'm trying to make: *There can be instances of too much information (TMI) in medical care!* According to the IOM, there are approximately 90 Million people in our country with "limited health literacy", particularly those with "lower socioeconomic status, limited education or limited English proficiency... ...the elderly and individuals with mental and physical disabilities." In turn, the Department of Health and Human Services (DHHS) has made it a priority to improve our country's health literacy. In principle, I think this is a worthy cause; one that will very likely help deliver patient care more effectively. The danger, as with all other topics in this book, stems from overcompensating by uncritically exposing the public to enormous amounts of complex information that is not relevant to their decision-making process, rather than staying within the boundaries of the basic construct of the patient-physician relationship (Figure 1-1). The premise used by the IOM and the DHHS to justify their proposals for improving health literacy begins with a listing of the tasks required from patients in the context of making medical decisions. Let's examine the reasonableness of these, one at a time:

1) <u>Evaluating information for credibility and quality</u>. Let me ask the reader a question: If you only had a basic proficiency of the English language, could you properly

appreciate Shakespeare or Byron? I doubt it! So, why is it that we are willing to expect that individuals without medical training should be able to assess how credible medical statements are, or the "quality" of medical information? I think this is an unrealistic expectation and I cannot help but wonder the potential ulterior motives for its inclusion. Think about it! Even for those of us with significant medical education and experience, evaluating the credibility of diagnostic and treatment information may sometimes be a daunting task, and one fraught with disagreements among professionals. So, how can we possibly expect that the medically uneducated or experienced can carry it out effectively? Perhaps the answer has to do with steering patients towards information that has been "approved" by "credible" organizations. Interestingly, a tour through one of these organizations' (i.e. American Academy of Neurology) patient education resources shows that the materials available are basically a lay interpretation of the "guidelines"; the consensus recommendations made by the *intelligentsia* by applying Evidence Based Medicine (EBM) rules. The message here is for patients to trust the information for sources such as this, almost as if their endorsement represents a seal of approval. Although I do not want to dwell on my criticisms of EBM (see Chapter 2), I submit that promoting health literacy and then controlling the type of information the public is to consider "credible" and of "quality" is manipulative and underhanded. It is no different than when Fidel Castro used to boast of the high percentage of literacy in the Cuban population, while the government controlled and approved the reading material available. Furthermore, I know from my daily interactions with patients, that they access all types of other information that is truly of poor quality, and cannot tell the difference. This often leads to extreme confusion and underscores my argument that it is simply ludicrous to think that most people should be able to assess the credibility and quality of medical information. Sooner or later they are going to have to trust the recommendations of the physician (Figure 1-1).

2) Analyzing relative risks and benefits. This task, although very reasonable, can be more difficult than suspected. It is at the heart of the use of *"informed consents"* for the performance of invasive and surgical procedures. I have no problem with providing patients with a list of the benefits and risks of any proposed course of action; in fact I do this on a daily basis. However, carrying out a balanced benefit vs. risk analysis in order to arrive at the best possible decision requires more than just attention to numbers. To illustrate, let's consider how patients approach the difference between risk *frequency* and risk *severity*. For example, the risk of accidentally perforating a cerebral aneurysm during endovascular treatment is very small; but the severity is huge! In other words, the chance of a problem arising is minimal but, if it does, the result is likely to be devastating! Both of these characteristics need to be taken into consideration when discussing the proposed procedure, but patients consistently have a hard time separating their respective impact. Moreover, by spewing long lists of risk percentages that may be considered "pertinent information", we may be creating a more confusing and counterproductive experience for the patient. Also, as we will cover in the next few pages, patients and families typically lack the prerequisite knowledge to properly

analyze the information and, sooner or later they are going to have to trust the recommendations of the physician (Figure 1-1).

3) Calculating dosages. This one is simply baffling. Patients have no need to calculate anything! Prescriptions already include appropriate dosages and I submit that it is downright dangerous for them to be given latitude to manipulate dosage schedules. To illustrate the potential problems, let us consider that most patients think that the amount of milligrams (mg) used in prescriptions is equivalent across different medications. So, patients who are used to the typical dose of rizatriptan (a drug commonly used to treat migraine headaches) being 10 mg commonly think that the equivalent typical dose of sumatriptan (a similar drug in the same class) of 100 mg is ten times stronger; it is not! So, when it comes to medication dosages, patients sooner or later are going to have to trust the recommendations of the physician (Figure 1-1).

4) Interpreting test results. Here is another example of uncritical thinking. In general, patients do not have the background and prerequisite knowledge to interpret results; they have to be interpreted for them. This is why, despite the fact that it is certainly their right to personally read the transcribed report of... ...let's say an MRI study, I usually discourage it because all it adds is confusion and additional irrelevant questions. Almost weekly I get to see a patient sent to me due to how a report reads! The typical scenario is that of a 65 year-old man who underwent an MRI at the request of his primary physician and both of them are baffled by a report that reads

something like *"prominent Virchow-Robin spaces"*. And so I have to sit in one of my examining rooms with a very frightened or concern patient because of his "Virchow-Robin spaces" and the seemingly ominous concern that they are prominent, and explain to him that this is... ...Normal! I contend that it is up to us to interpret the meaning of test results for the patients, translating technobabble into terms that have meaning and allow the patient to use the information appropriately. Thus, when it comes to interpreting test results, the patients sooner or later are going to have to trust the recommendations of the physician (Figure 1-1).

5) <u>Locating health information</u>. Actually, I think this is very similar to #1 above. It requires critical thinking not only to decide on the credibility of medical information, but also to assess the various sources. Otherwise, the same problem we pointed out operates here: being at the mercy of organizations considered credible by default, whether justifiably so or not.

So, it seems like the tasks that have been assigned to patients based on their health literacy have an unrealistic trait to them. Moreover, it seems that no matter how literate the patient is, he is going to have to trust the physician for an interpretation of the information and advice about its applicability.

In addition of the comments I have made above, a closer look at the published information on health literacy reveals a not so straightforward conceptual scaffold. It is difficult, when reviewing information from the IOM, to know where general literacy ends and literacy specific for medicine begins. In fact, the most important review of the existing literature on the subject clearly addresses general literacy (i.e. reading ability) and its impact on healthcare. Thus, if the argument is that a literate patient is a better patient, I would say... ...Duh! However, if the argument is that a patient who has more health-related information is a better patient, then I would say... ...It depends on the quality of the information and how able is the individual to incorporate it into his own knowledge level, experience and priorities. This is, in my view, a more important aspect of patient education. In the next few pages, I want to paint a picture abut the current climate on educating patients, including realistic priorities, reasonable expectations, and the downgrading effect of several cultural changes that pervade current communication between physicians and patients.

It used to be, following our original basic construct of the physician–patient relationship (Figure 1–1) that in any clinical situation the expert party was the physician. Therefore, patients and their families would seek the advice of their physician, and listened attentively to the explanations and instructions in order to be able to follow them to the letter. Then, the physician would offer to answer any questions and would do so gladly. In those days, it was not unusual for the following conversation to take place:

> PATIENT: *"I have a stupid question"*
>
> PHYSICIAN: *"There are no stupid questions, so go ahead and ask"*

This interaction was followed by the patient asking the question that he had in mind, and the physician addressing it as best as he could. The reader is likely to recognize that the key element in the exchange captioned above is the innocent curiosity of the patient regarding the information being sought. Through the years, many of us encountered such a similar situation and were more than happy to accommodate the inquisitiveness of the patient and to spend time covering the relevant information that filled the knowledge gap. The key to answering these questions was to keep the answers in simple and understandable terms, avoiding technobabble, and trying to promote basic understanding of very complex processes by people with little knowledge foundation of the subject at hand. I have always thought it was important to avoid "labeling" conditions due to patients having a tendency to latch on to terms and, sort of, getting "stuck" on them in such ways that became hindrances and obstacles to their own care. For example, it is not uncommon at present to experience an encounter similar to the following:

> PHYSICIAN: *"So, what brings you to see us?"*

> PATIENT: *"I have neuropathy!"*

Following this answer, I cannot help myself and I ask:

> PHYSICIAN: *"Maybe you can tell me your symptoms and I can make my own diagnosis..."*

Unfortunately, this example is not the exception but the rule. Typically, patients who show up using terms such as *"neuropathy"*, *"dementia"* or *"TIA"*, learned these either from another physician who uses medical terminology uncritically, or from a non-medical source. The truth is that we practice medicine at a time when anyone who has access to the Internet has the audacity to have a medical opinion. Moreover, they do not have the sense to keep it to themselves, but rather they share their opinions openly, as if having acquired them online guarantees their correctness. They even dare to show up in our clinic using medical terminology freshly learned online; failing to realize that not only they *do not impress us, but they also appear foolish!* You think I am being harsh? Well, let me place my criticism in perspective. Imagine that I were to engage in a conversation with one of the scientists from the *U.S. Space and Rocket Center* in Huntsville, Alabama. Now imagine that I decided to introduce into the conversation all sorts of rocketry terminology I had learned in one session of cybersurf; for example, *"igniters"*, or *"total impulse power"*. Do you really think these rocket scientists would be impressed by my conceitedness? I doubt it! The same is true in our clinic! So we rather have patients keep their diagnostic and therapeutic opinions to themselves.

Nevertheless, it does not matter what we want. The current culture is one of gathering information, irrespective of relevance, under the premise that more is better, and share it with others whether they like it or not. Moreover, the different tone of the current inquisitorial exchange between patients and physicians stems from changes in attitude related to the sense of entitlement discussed in the previous chapter. In turn, those attitudinal changes include a partial or complete mistrust of the physician, a self-centered outlook regarding the "right to know" (this is not so unfair when the patient himself is the one asking questions, but it becomes a real problem when every member of a large family has the same attitude and wants to hear information directly), and more importantly the delusion that spending 20 minutes in front of the computer doing an Internet search provides anyone without a medical background with a fair understanding of the clinical issues at hand. Therefore, the interactions between patients and families with the physicians are not uncommonly highlighted by suspicion, skepticism, mistrust, disrespect and downright arrogance. Does this seem like a recipe for good medicine? I dare say no!

And so, it has become increasingly frequent for the patient to approach the physician with questions that are based not on his own innocent curiosity, but rather on other information acquired from a variety of sources. The most frequent of these sources is the one I have mentioned elsewhere in the book as *"The Advisors"*: Neighbors, coworkers, family members, or even friends of friends who speak with unjustified authority about subjects they have experienced, heard about, or seen in television, usually by viewing reruns of *House* or *Grey's Anatomy*. They advise patients and families with absolutely no shame or remorse, not even considering the possibility that they simply do not have a clue as to what they are talking about. As I was growing up, we used to refer to this frame of mind as *"hearing bells but not knowing where the church is!"* Sometimes, even other professionals become part of The Advisors. Just today, a young patient of mine came for follow up to clinic and shared with me how her physical therapist had suggested that she might need additional MRI studies for diagnosis. Obviously, this got her concerned and doubtful of how thorough our previous imaging evaluation had been. The truth is that she does not need any more testing but the out-of-turn commentary resulted in the need for additional time and energy expenditure on my part, and not to say the anxiety generated in the patient and her family. So, the frequent interference of individuals whispering advice in the ears of our patients is yet another downgrading aspect of the current healthcare climate.

Nevertheless, as bad as the influence of The Advisors seems to be, it does not come close to that of the ubiquitous Internet searches carried out looking for the answers. I can assure you that this problem, if anything, continues to get worse. Patients and families actually think that they can surf the web and recognize reliable information from trash, or relevant information from that which has nothing to do with their problem. Not too long ago, for example, a young girl with what was clearly a psychiatric disorder came to my clinic with her family convinced that she had *"ballismus"*, a fairly rare movement disorder. Competing with the information superhighway is often exhausting and unproductive because not only we have to provide a sensible diagnosis but also undo a whole cadre of misconceptions. The worst manifestation of this behavior is the practice of bringing Internet printouts to clinic to show them to the physician, a custom I consider disrespectful, shortsighted, and presumptuous!

If my words appear to be too harsh, I would invite you to consider the following: The next time you are taking a trip in a commercial airliner, as you enter the airplane, before turning right to take your seat, try turning left and telling the captain that you have an Internet search printout that explains how to fly this particular aircraft, and that you would like very much for him to review it. Sounds crazy? Well, in my view, not any crazier than patients bringing Internet printouts to my clinic and pretending to educate me on a subject that I have been handling for over three decades. Typically, I either do not look at such printouts or casually decline to do so. Occasionally, when dealing with some of the most obnoxious individuals, I have simply thrown them in the trashcan so there is no doubt as to what I think of such behavior. The latter response is usually followed by an expression of astonishment on their part, and then an inquisitive looks accompanied by a question: *"Why did you do that?"* My answer to such questions is invariably another question: *"Why do you feel the need to insult me?"* Now he really looks astonished! The conversation usually ends after I express to them how insulting I find his audacity to think that he could find information more relevant, let alone reliable, than I could provide about the clinical subject at hand.

The problem of Internet searches and how they impact the patient–physician relationship goes further. They influence the attitude of the patient during the clinical encounter. At a time when most of us wish they were listening to our opinion and advice (after all this is the reason why they came to see us), they are not doing so because they are too busy thinking about all of the ideas generated by their Internet searches. In fact, if one looks closely, it is possible to see that within microseconds of the end of our explanation of their condition, diagnosis, and proposed treatment, they eagerly begin to bring out questions based upon their half-ass knowledge, as if we had not said a word. It is at this time that the interaction we showed earlier could be rewritten as follows:

PATIENT: *"I have a stupid question"*

PHYSICIAN: *" Well keep it to yourself. We do not answer stupid questions on Tuesday."*

But that would be too rude of a response. In all fairness, the patients and their families are simply following the cues of a system that has progressively built a sense of entitlement that includes the misperception of themselves as critical medical thinkers. This flawed culture does not recognize that it is practically impossible for anyone without medical education to correctly assess the veracity, relevance, applicability and actuality of pieces of information acquired through an Internet search; clearly an unregulated source of information. The logic of such behavior is clearly missing. Furthermore, most reasonable and experienced physicians I know couldn't care less what the patient or her family found in the Internet during one of their cyber escapades.

In summary, patient education is a very important variable in the delivery of medical care. In order for the fundamental construct of the physician-patient relationship to work effectively, however, the education of patients needs to have a realistic design. At present, the position of the government and its cronies regarding "Health Literacy" is somewhat puzzling, with background information often referring to general literacy instead. In this context, the entire subject seems to be based on the assumption that patients must carry out a certain set of "tasks" as part of their role in healthcare delivery. A closer look at these reveals their inappropriate assignment as patients' responsibilities, and shows that they cannot replace their trust in physicians' advice. Despite the need for *real* education, patients seeking information from unreliable sources such as friends and the Internet characterize the current climate. This translates into patients often interfering with clinical encounters by inappropriately introducing unwanted and erroneous information. Generally, this behavior is part of the entitlement attitude seen in other aspects of patient interactions. Yes, medical literacy is important, but overdoing it is liable to cause more confusion and will likely be counterproductive.

20

Treatment Complications

"Nichol's 4th Law:
Avoid any action with an unacceptable outcome!"

George E. Nichols
Engineer and Project Manager
NASA Jet Propulsion Laboratory

A quote whose original source I have never found reads *"the only operators that deny having complications either have not performed enough procedures, or they are lying!"* Anyone who has practiced medicine for any length of time should be able to assert that this is a truism. Alas, even the best of physician runs into complications of the treatment prescribed, to no fault of his own, without a hint of negligence, and despite his decision having been the most reasonable under the clinical circumstances in which he made it. Treatment complications can be categorized as technical (i.e. resulting from either procedures going astray), or medical (i.e. the product of medications side effect), both constituting unintended consequences of the physician's actions. In addition, complications can range from very mild and completely reversible, to disabling or even fatal. They are a ubiquitous and invisible threat to the well being of our patients, and the successful outcome of any therapeutic strategy, and loom as the proverbial *Sword of Damocles* over the patient-physician interactions. Despite their negative connotation, they are natural variables of the clinical equation, and their existence should not be considered any more artificial than that of the shadows created by the light. In the next few pages, I would like to discuss the role that treatment complications play in the day-to-day practice of medicine, as well as their relationship to the downgrading process of the healthcare system. I would also like the reader to become aware of the fact that it is impossible to separate the intended benefits of any treatment from its potential risks, both known and imponderable.

So, how do we navigate the sea of decision-making while safely avoiding the obstacles along our path; those that are likely to result in a poor outcome? In my view, the only way to do so is to embrace a very realistic view of what medicine is, and what is not! Earlier in the book, I made reference to several very important concepts that need to be integrated in our understanding of the role that potential complications must play in our decisions about medical treatment. Perhaps the most important of them all is the concept of *Quality of Life*, as the most important outcome variable of the treatment we offer patients. As I have pointed out, everyone is going to die sooner or later and the main goal of medicine is not to prolong the heart beating indiscriminately but to prevent untimely and unnecessary deaths, while at the same time optimizing the quality of the life of the patient. It is within the framework of this concept that we must analyze the benefits and risks of treatment, if we are to derive a realistic conclusion about what course of treatment is worthwhile following, and which one must be abandoned. In looking at this subject from the point of view of promoting quality of life, it becomes an inescapable fact that *only the patient has the ability to decide on his own what quality of life means for him*! I think I emphasized the significance of this point very clearly in my concluding remarks about the true meaning of Evidence Based Medicine (EBM). In particular, the fact that the third "pillar" of EBM refers to the values of the patient and how he chooses to apply those to the decision-making process relative to his medical care. Thus, it seems that we have come full circle and we begin to see the importance of returning to the fundamental core values of the practice of medicine. Once we accept this more realistic paradigm, it is possible to recognize the strategies more likely to bring us closer to truly having patients provide the so-called *"Informed Consent"*.

In this context, we should parenthetically continue our discussion by first addressing how our construct applies to the assessment of invasive procedures used for diagnostic or therapeutic purposes. Although clearly every procedure has its own intended benefits and potential risks, we can group them in categories based upon the relationship between those two variables (Figure 20-1). In doing so, we can theoretically assess any procedure and have it fit somewhere in the grid provided, as a starting point in our quest for a reasonable analysis of benefit vs. risks for a given clinical situation. Ideally, a procedure that is very likely to benefit the patient would be much better off if it could be placed in the right lowermost square of the grid. This would mean that the benefit that is intended by performing this procedure is accompanied by a significantly low risk and makes the decision to proceed a *no-brainer!* Conversely, should the intended benefit to the patient be relatively small (i.e. left uppermost square), a procedure that carries a potentially high risk could be withheld with similar degree of certainty. This sounds fairly straightforward, doesn't it? Unfortunately, it is not so simple because of multiple other variables that need to be considered and that make the placement of any procedure into our proposed grid very often a challenging task. Let's walk through some of these:

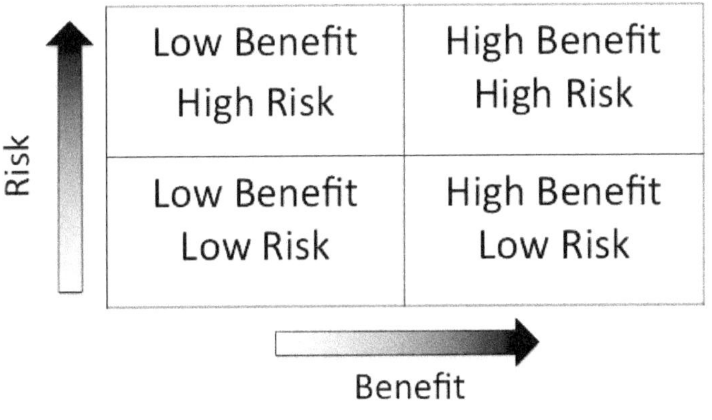

Figure 20-1
Benefit vs. Risk Grid

1) <u>Procedural heterogeneity</u>. Despite the fact that nearly all explicit procedures are based on the same blueprint, variations occur based upon schools of thought, educational programs, and local medical culture. Therefore, it is important to recognize that what works in an academic New York hospital may not be comparable to what happens in a rural hospital in Mississippi. For years, we have witnessed how the surgical style of specialists who underwent postgraduate education under certain

luminary surgeons oftentimes is at odds with that of individuals who worked under the tutelage of someone else halfway across the world. This is, in fact, not uncommon and I have witnessed it firsthand in the graduates of our fellowship program, whose style of practice has been to a great degree shaped by having worked with us day in and day out for several years.

2) Operator's expertise. This concept must also be exposed and discussed because it is not a common subject of dialog, particularly when people who are obsessed with EBM fail to recognize it as the second "pillar" of that discipline. For years now, as I lectured on various interventional topics, I have consistently hammered the concept that *"good equipment is not a substitute for good technique!"* There is absolutely no way to argue against the idea that not every operator has the same skills or experience and, therefore, even using the same blueprint of a procedure there are likely to be differences in outcomes based upon the operator's technique. But expertise does not only include technical skills; it also encompasses *clinical judgment.* This is the ability to decide when and if a procedure is necessary; for whom, and what are the hurdles that predictably can negatively alter the outcome. If we embrace the concept discussed in Chapter 19 in reference to Health Literacy, as it applies to the fact that eventually patients will have to trust the advice of a physician, then clinical judgment is *sine qua non* for an optimal outcome. Along my career, I have taught and worked guided by several very important rules, one of them being that *"the less clear the indication the more likely the complication!"* At the end of the day, without clinical judgment, most skillful operators are

bound to get themselves recurrently in trouble during the performance of procedures that were not very well planned or simply unnecessary.

3) Technologic advances. I think it is important to point out that, despite all the government interventions, technology in our country has advanced at a very rapid pace. Such advancement has resulted in the introduction of increasingly effective equipment for the performance of numerous procedures. For example, in my specialty we now have balloons and stents that can be delivered to the brain arteries with ease and speed, a fact that was not true when I started performing interventions in the early 1990's. Therefore, it is incumbent on every operator to be familiar with newer technologies that not only can facilitate procedures, but that can actually change the benefit vs. risk analysis itself.

4) Environmental support. Operators do not perform procedures in a vacuum. They require the participation of an entire cadre of people that support them, both administratively and practically. Therefore, it is important to recognize that the most brilliant and capable of operators may not be able to complete the same procedures within environments that are not suitable for such a feat. For example, also in my field of endeavor, angiographic equipment and the people who operate it must be of at least sufficient sophistication to allow the smooth performance of very complex interventions (e.g. treating a cerebral aneurysm using a single plane x-ray equipment is twice as difficult, and takes twice as long, than doing so in a dual plane system). Curiously, sometimes the environmental support structure

> wrongfully replaces the operator himself. This is the reason why there is such a mystique for patients to go to *"Mayo Clinic"*; or for patients in South America to commonly speak of going to have their open-heart surgery in *"Houston"*. As you can see, it almost becomes irrelevant to these people who are they going to see, so long as they are treated within an environment they perceive as the best available for the problem. I can assure the reader, after having visited or worked in some of these places whose names are repeated as if they meant *Mecca*, that their importance as good support systems is real, although not primordial.

And so, the task of placing any one procedure into the benefit vs. risk grid (Figure 20-1) can indeed become a formidable task. Once again, it will be the strength of the physician–patient relationship that will allow the most effective way for the decision-making process to evolve into the best outcome for the individual. This illustrates that the "informed consent process" goes well beyond the listing of numerous possible things that can go astray regarding a procedure, and the odds that they will. For it to be realistic and just to the patient, it has to include an interaction whereby the patient's values guide the physician's judgment into making the soundest of advices in order to maximize the opportunity for the best outcome.

Let's turn our attention now to a bigger and more common problem: *Medication side effects!* It should be no secret to the reader by now that, in my opinion, physicians can be more dangerous with a prescription pad than with a scalpel! All you have to do is follow my description of polypharmacy (Chapter 6) to understand my concerns about the ease with which we seem to administer drugs to patients, while breaking fundamental rules of prescription practice, and failing to take into account the complexity of drug interactions and their potentially harmful effects. Unlike my other criticisms about the position of the government agencies and their surrogates pertinent to other topics, I think there is an underestimation on their part of the problem at hand. If we were to construct a decision flowchart relative to the administration of medications based upon an encounter between a physician and a patient, the odds of the

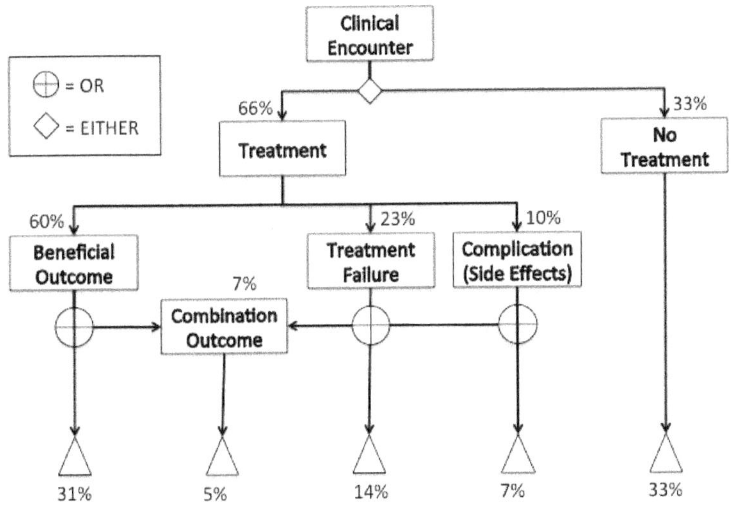

Figure 20-2
Projected Outcomes from Medication Use
(Modified from Ernst & Grizzle)

various outcomes of such an interaction are illustrated in Figure 20-2. Interestingly, the existing literature is quite consistent on the subject, and mimics some of the data I acquired in my clinic and shared with you in Chapter 6 (although I think it underrepresents the problem). Historically, the odds that a patient will be given a pill following an encounter with a physician approximate 2 to 1 (i.e. about 66%). Once this pill is taken, there is less than a 60% chance that it will produce a beneficial outcome devoid of any unwanted side effects. The remaining patients will have partial benefit, no benefit, only side effects, or a combination of these. Therefore, just like with invasive procedures, the decision to administer a patient a pill must include some form of benefit vs. risk analysis. Most of us carry this out in a discipline and almost obsessive fashion; but most of us are hesitant about prescribing medications in general unless such an analysis clearly favors the benefit to the patient. In reference to my original comments about polypharmacy, it is self evident that a benefit vs. risk analysis of prescription practices becomes increasingly difficult and inaccurate when many medications are present concurrently, and their interactions become less predictable.

Does this mean that, before prescribing a medication for a patient, we have to list for them all of the *potential side effects* they could experience? Personally, I think this is a somewhat ridiculous practice and I would like to try to make a case for my opinion. First of all, we already agreed that there is a large percentage of the population that, due to their health illiteracy, has difficulty understanding all of the information that is given to them. So, what makes us think that adding a laundry list of potential side effects is going to clarify things for them? In my experience, such a practice leads to nothing more than confusion and suggestion for the patient. Second, what difference does it make? As I have repeatedly noted, with a few exceptions that must be dealt differently, the overwhelming majority of side effects from medications are *"potential"* and may never occur. Therefore, this bogus practice of "educating" patients on every single potential side effect that they may never have, serves absolutely no practical purpose. This is particularly true when we consider the fact that the majority of the side effects that may develop are transient and bound to disappear once the drug is discontinued. I beg the reader's indulgence in not underestimating the day-to-day impact of how side effect "education" is handled in our country. As I have mentioned earlier, none the least of the problems is that, irrespective of what we tell the patients, the pharmacists are very likely to engage in a dialogue that many times results in the patient not taking the medications prescribed and essentially wasting the time he spent in our clinic. On the other hand, despite the fact that I disagree with the Institute of Medicine (IOM) assessment of this as a "crisis", it is true that medication prescription errors occur. Largely speaking, however, this subject does not typically apply to side effects and their occurrence, and should have no bearing on our assessment of the subject.

So, what can we do to make the patients aware of the potential negative consequences of taking the medication, without suggesting to them what those will be, or confusing them with unnecessary information? My answer is simple: *Logic!* If we use rules of engagement that are based on logic and reason, I submit that we can protect the patients without overwhelming them with irrelevant data. As an example, here's what I recommend:

1) <u>In general, start only one medication at a time</u>. With only a few exceptional situations, there is absolutely no earthly reason for patients to be given more than one brand-new medication at a time. By breaking this rule, we expose the patient to an increased level of unpredictability of side effects and a possible negative outcome.

2) <u>Reassess promptly after every new prescription</u>. Physicians who start a patient on a brand-new

medication and give them a follow-up appointment three months later constantly baffle me. I find this practice not only unreasonable but also dangerous. If the patient is to start taking a new medication, the most reasonable thing to do is to see him again in a week or two (depending upon the medication), so we can reassess the resulting benefit and potential side effects.

3) Instruction: *"Anything new warrants earlier reassessment!"* Instead of providing patients with a long list of potential side effects, their education should be a lot simpler. Essentially, the patient should be taught that if they feel differently after starting to take a brand-new medication, chances are that this is the result of the drug itself. If such difference is significantly bothersome, they need to come in earlier than scheduled for reassessment.

As you can see, what I propose follows the KISS (Keep It Simple Stupid) principle. I submit that we have a greater chance for patient compliance with these instructions if we make them easy to understand and easy to follow. Unfortunately, as I said earlier, not a week goes by in which some pharmacist somewhere sabotages a perfectly good plan of mine. That said, I like to make a comment about the exceptional situations I mentioned earlier. There are medications that have inherent potential side effects that are either *irreversible* or *unequivocal*. The former are considerably worse than the latter but any of these two groups probably warrants a deeper analysis of the benefits vs. the risks, and a more explicit discussion with the patient.

Lucky for us and the patients, scientific advances are now available to assess each and every patient's genetic construct in an attempt to predict how they're going to react to a specific medication. *Pharmacogenomics* is the science that studies the relationship between the patient's genetic make up and his response to specific drugs; the genetic variations that cause differences in drug response among individuals. Presently, it is possible by a simple oral swab to carry out this type of assessment in every patient prior to prescribing medications (http://naturalmolecular.com), helping us understand and predict with greater clarity the intended beneficial effect and potential side effects that *this* patient specifically has for *this* drug.

In summary, treatment complications are a reality. The ability to carry out either an invasive procedure, or to prescribe a medication without causing more harm than good is at the core of good medicine. Although the ideal procedures are those with great benefit and low risk, and the most undesirable ones are those with great risk and little benefit, the fact is that the overwhelming majority of them are difficult to gauge without realistically looking at a series of variables that will impact how procedures are planned and carried out. At the end of the day, and whether anyone likes it or not, it will be necessary for the patient to trust the advice of the physician regarding certain procedures. More commonly, however, the problem of overprescribing medications in our country carries with it a significant consequence in terms of side effect production. Despite this, it seems unreasonable to attempt to have patients memorize lists of potential side effects that may never occur. Alternatively, simpler and more practical approaches must be sought and utilized in clinical medicine. Finally, it will be important for other "healthcare providers" to refrain from interfering by introducing their own professional agenda.

21

Generic Medications

"The most dangerous untruths are truths slightly distorted."

Georg C. Lichtenberg
German Scientist and Satirist
(1742 - 1799)

It is said that if someone sells you a $1,000 diamond ring for $10, chances are you own a diamond not worth $0.50. Generic medications fit this aphorism quite well. One of the most downgrading trends in our healthcare system is that of pushing generic medications onto patients because of their lower cost. The push comes from insurance carriers that refuse to pay for brand name medications, pharmacists who make a larger profit margin by selling generic versions of a drug and, or course, the government. Yes; the government! Through the years, it has been the Food and Drug Administration (FDA) the one regulating and enforcing any and all legal aspects pertinent to prescription medications, especially generics. In the next few pages I want to review this topic and its impact of its use on the current healthcare culture, paying particular attention to critical aspects that are seldom part of the discussions about our downgraded system.

Let's begin by taking a historical tour of how drugs are approved in our country, and how we got to the present status of the use of generic medications. The first governmental move to exert some control of medication-related issues was the Pure Food and Drug Act of 1906. This law provided federal inspection of meat products and forbade the manufacture, sale or transportation of poisonous "patent medicines". The latter were those sold with heavy promotion as prodigious cures (e.g. snake oil liniments), but did nothing of what was promised. Parenthetically, the term "patent" is misused in association with them since they were not actually *patented.* In any case, the act was the result of then President Theodore Roosevelt supporting the progressive movement claiming for more government-based protection of consumers. It required that certain drugs, including alcohol, cocaine, heroin, morphine, and cannabis (i.e. marihuana) be correctly labeled with contents and dosages instead of being sold as patent medicines. Interestingly, all of these continued to be legally available without prescription, so long as they were properly labeled. Although at first the act was mainly concerned with labeling, after some time there were efforts to outlaw products that were not safe, followed by the intent to outlaw products that were safe but not effective. As a historical curiosity, it was this legislation that resulted in Coca-Cola having to reduce the amount of caffeine in its formula.[9] As a result of the Coca-Cola litigation, the act was amended in 1912 to include caffeine among the list of habit-forming substances that must

---

[9] Caffeine had replaced cocaine as the main stimulant in Coca-Cola in 1903

be specified in labels. The Pure Food and Drug Act of 1906 heralded the creation of the FDA in 1927; an event that resulted from the reorganization of the Bureau of Chemistry into the Food, Drug, and Insecticide Administration, and the Bureau of Chemistry and Soils.

The next chapter in our story is the Food, Drug and Cosmetic Act of 1938 (FD&C), signed into law by then President Franklin D. Roosevelt, and which conferred the FDA the authority to oversee the safety of food, drugs, and cosmetics. Its introduction was precipitated by the death of over 100 patients from poisoning from diethylene glycol having been used as a diluent to make sulfanilamide into an elixir. This act has been amended numerous times, the most important for our discussion being the Drug Price Competition and Patent Restoration Act of 1984. However, before we address the latter, allow me to make a few comments about two important amendments to the FD&C: a) The FD&C Amendment of 1962, and b) The Medical Device Regulation Act of 1976, with its Section 510(k). The significance of the former is that it included statutes pertinent to requiring proof-of-efficacy for the approval of drugs. Until then, only proof-of-safety was necessary. The latter is remarkable because it represents a device approval process somewhat similar to that currently in place for generic medications. The original FD&C only allowed the FDA to remove adulterated or mis-branded medical devices. Please note that, in 1938, medical devices included relatively simple instruments such as stethoscopes and scalpels. However, by the early 1970s, a government commission had determined that more than 700 deaths and 10,000 injuries had resulted from defective medical devices (e.g. heart valves, pacemakers); this set the stage for the introduction of this amendment. Among its statutes, the act requires device manufacturers to notify the FDA at least 90 days in advance of their intent to market a medical device. This is known as Premarket Notification (PMN) or 510(k), and it allows the FDA to determine whether the device is "substantially equivalent" [10] to a device that has already undergone Premarket Approval (PMA), the standard pathway to bring any new device to market. Devices that reach the market via the 510(k) process are not considered "approved" but rather "cleared" to be sold in the United States. However, recent publications suggest that, of the devices recalled by the FDA because they could cause serious health problems or death, the great majority (more than 70%) were devices cleared via the 510(k) process. So much for "substantially equivalent"!

This brings us to the Drug Price Competition and Patent Restoration Act of 1984, also known the "Hatch-Waxman Act". This is the federal law that established the current system for generic medications and it is named after representative Henry A. Waxman (D-CA) and senator Orrin Hatch (R-UT). The ideas behind this piece of legislation began during President Jimmy Carter's Administration, when in 1978 he launched a major domestic policy review of industrial innovation. The results of this included a recommendation for patent term restoration for pharmaceuticals in order to compensate them for the time lost in regulatory review. For drugs approved prior to 1962, generic versions could be approved with a "paper" new drug application (NDA). The latter was based merely on published scientific or medical literature, and so a generic manufacturer could get a drug approved by simply showing the existence of specialized publications that endorsed the safety of the chemical in question. After 1962, congressional

---

[10] Remember this term because it is at the core of our discussion

records show that generic producing companies where unwilling to spend time and money to produce generic versions of approximately 150 drugs that the time where off-patent. Moreover, there were only 15 "paper NDAs" for generic versions of post–1962 drugs. Picking up where Carter left it, President Reagan's Cabinet Council on Commerce and Trade supported the proposal noted above, and which became a bill that passed the Senate but failed to pass at the House of Representatives. At that time,

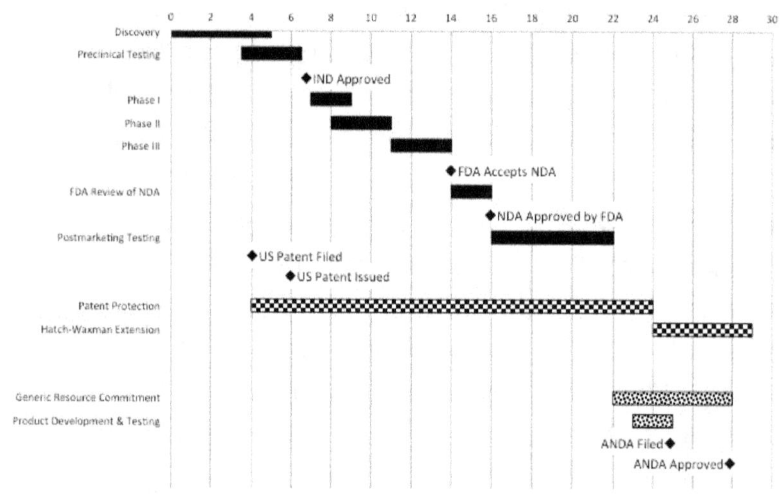

Figure 21-1
New Drug Approval, Patents & Generic Approval Timeline

Congressman Waxman took on the issue and was instrumental in adding the drug price competition part, complicating the bill substantially. Following the enactment of the Hatch-Waxman Act, the Uruguay Round Agreements Act (resulting from the negotiations that led to the creation of the World Trade Organization) provided that any drug with a patent in effect (or a patent application pending) on June, 1995 would receive a term of 20 years from the time of filing or 17 years from the time of granting, whichever was longer. Although such a resolution may seem fair by providing the pharmaceutical company that developed the drug with significant amount of time to recover their investment, the current timeline for bringing a new drug into the market essentially utilizes most of that time (Figure 21-1). This is an important aspect of the whole process; one that I will cover further in the next few pages.

A closer study of the Hatch–Waxman Act shows that, forsooth, its Title I contains the drug price competition part, specifically authorizes Abbreviated New Drug Applications (ANDA), and expressly forbids the FDA from asking anything other than bioavailability studies for the approval of generic medications through the ANDA process. The latter represents the current mechanism by which generic drugs enter the market (Figure 21-1). Thus, when a company files an ANDA, it is required to issue one of four certifications, currently known as paragraphs I, II, III and IV, as follow:

1) <u>The drug has not been patented</u> (I).

2) <u>The patent has already expired</u> (II).

3) <u>The date on which the patent will expire, and the intent not to market the generic drug until after such date</u> (III).

4) <u>The patent is not infringed, or is invalid</u> (IV).

Title 35 of the United States Code includes the patent term restoration part of the Act of Hatch-Waxman. This is also shown in Figure 21-1, illustrating how a pioneer company (i.e. the originator of the brand-name drug) receives an extension term equal to one half of the time of the investigational new drug (IND) period. Moreover, the maximum extension of total market exclusivity granted is five years, and the total market exclusivity time cannot exceed 14 years. Interestingly, the lengths of the exclusivity periods represent completely arbitrary and bureaucratic numbers, without any scientific or reasonable foundation. What? The government being arbitrary? *Please say it ain't so!* To make matters worse, the act includes a prohibition by which the pioneer drug company must exercise due diligence in order to achieve a patent term restoration; a provision that has never been used! The result is that the day after the patent expires, generic drugs supposed to be "substantially equivalent" (remember I told you about this term earlier in the chapter!) become available in pharmacies and are ready to be dispensed to patients.

Next, let's focus our discussion on the generic medications themselves; what they are and what they are not. Let me start by making a categorical statement: *It is my opinion that generic drugs are never the same as the brand name counterpart!* I would like to begin this part of the discussion by referring the reader to the government's case for generic drugs, illustrated by statements that can easily be found in the FDA website (www.FDA.gov), and I list here together with my criticisms and points of view:

1) "FDA requires generic drugs to have the same active ingredient, strength, dosage form, a route of administration as the brand name drug." On the surface, this particular statement seems to have a self-evident reasonableness. It stresses the fact that the generic version of a pill, for example, must have the same medication amount than the original brand-name pill. So, the question that comes to mind is: *if the two pills are identical, what need is there to do any of the bioavailability*

testing that is required? There does not seem to be a reasonable answer unless one takes into account the fact that there are indeed differences and that the law allows these, as we will see below.

2) "The generic manufacturer must prove its drug is the same (bioequivalent) as the brand-name drug." This statement constitutes the most important in our discussion since it represents the epicenter of a deception that results in patients often being treated with inferior medications that endanger their lives, just to shift profits from one group to another. It clearly is in complete contradiction to my opinion stated earlier, but only one of the two positions can be correct. Interestingly, the FDA itself admits that the drugs are not the same by additional explanations: *"Any generic drug modeled after a single brand name drug must perform approximately the same in the body as the brand-name drug. There will always be a slight, but not medically important, level of natural variability..."* Different tune, isn't it? First we are told that the two drugs are the same, but later the qualifier "approximately" is utilized to indicate the variance between the two. Through the clever utilization of different terminology, the government gets away with pushing a cost agenda; one that we will also discuss later in the book. Let's concentrate on this variability between a generic drug and the brand-name medication is supposed to replace. If you look carefully at the original statement made by the government they imply that their definition of "the same" is that they are "bioequivalent", which essentially means that the amount of active ingredient in the blood over a period of time is similar between the two drugs being compared. Unfortunately, a

detail that is not commonly discussed is that the FDA will approve a generic drug if its bioavailability is plus-or-minus 20% of the brand name (Figure 21-2). Twenty percent is a significant margin, particularly for drugs that have a very narrow therapeutic range (i.e. those medications in which small variability of dosages carry significant impact on the care the patient). Let me expand on this point and try to explain it in greater detail since its importance is crucial for understanding the downgrading

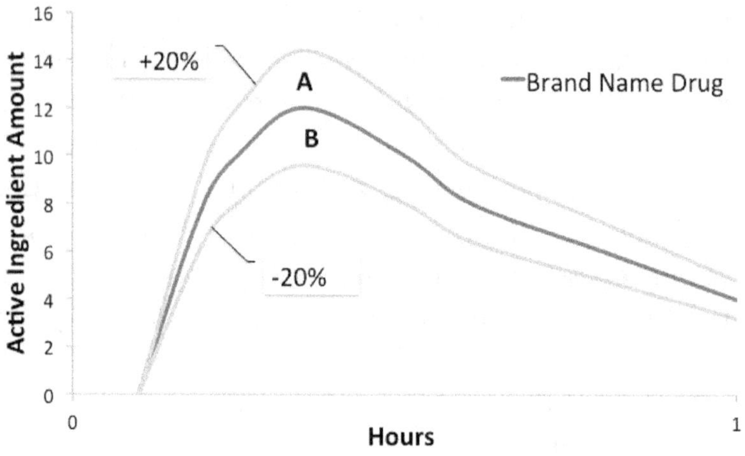

Figure 21-2
Bioavailability and FDA Allowances for Generic Drugs

effect that generic medications can have on medical treatments. In Figure 21-2 we see the bioavailability curve of a brand name drug, superimposed on which we have bioavailability curves that are plus-or- minus 20%. Since we already covered the fact that these are comparisons of medications with the same amount of active ingredient, it follows that a patient whose generic medication places him in the Plus 20% (A, in the figure), is more likely to have potential side effects from the same dose of medication. Conversely, a patient whose generic medication places him in the Minus 20% (B, in the figure) is likely to have less of the intended benefit of the medication. To make matters even worse, there are numerous generic versions of certain drugs; a fact that the FDA expresses as an advantage for better pricing due to competition. However, they fail to recognize that different generic versions of the same drug may have different bioavailability curves and, therefore, every time the patient gets his prescription refilled he may be getting a totally different product. This problem is not too bad in cases where the medication has a wide therapeutic range or those in which the consequences of being off by 20% are not life-threatening; for example, thyroid supplementation. There are numerous generic versions of this but, since most patients' thyroid function is monitored during treatment, the physician can adjust dosing without significant risk for the patient. However, if the drug has a narrow therapeutic range (e.g. seizure medications) or if the consequences of being off by 20% can be devastating (e.g. stroke prevention drugs), I submit that using generic medications is a recipe for a catastrophe. The impact of these problems in the practice of neurology has been enormous. Two examples come to mind: Keppra® and Plavix®! The former is a very effective seizure control medication of which, by my last count, there are over 25 different generic versions. The latter, a very effective drug for stroke prevention, became generic earlier this year. There are already 9 different generic versions of it and, since their introduction we have already had 10 cases of patients who suffered strokes after they were switched from the brand name to one of the generics.

3) "All manufacturing, packaging, and testing sites must pass the same quality standards as those of brand-name drugs." The FDA boasts that the fact that generic medications have a lower price does not mean that they are inferior. However, the assumption that a bioequivalence data represent an effective surrogate for the safety and efficacy of generic drugs cannot be defended. Clearly, they're not the same medication as the brand name they mimic and so, it is impossible to believe that the manufacturing quality of these different drugs is identical. They are clearly cheaper, about 80-85% less on the average, and the FDA claims that generic medications saved $158 billion in 2010. They also note that the manufacturers of generic medications can sell the product at a lower cost because they do not have to invest in the convoluted process of being the first one approved (i.e. NDA and IND). Although this is true, there is more to this issue, as you will see later in this chapter.

4) "Many generic drugs are made in the same manufacturing plants as the brand-name drugs." What is this supposed to mean? Are we to understand that using the same equipment, in the same location, guarantees the same quality? First of all, it is only in a minority of cases that this takes place. Second, since we established that the generic version of the brand name is different, there have to be some disparities in how the two are manufactured, regardless of where this takes place.

At this time, I think it is fair for us to refocus the topic of our discussion on issues of cost. As we mentioned earlier, there is no doubt that generic versions of brand-name drugs are cheaper. However, if you remember our previous discussion regarding the relationship between cost, quality and value (Chapter 8), it should be clear to you that there is an optimal price for a drug that serves a certain purpose and at which it is of optimal value to the patient. It should also be implicit in such an understanding that to consider the cost of medications, without taking into account their quality, makes no medical or economic sense. Based upon the discussion so far, we can state that on the average it takes approximately 12 years and over $350 million to get a new drug from the laboratory onto the pharmacy shelf. If you apply some of the information that I have shared with you earlier, you will quickly come to the realization that a company must have revenues in the range of $25 to $40 million per year of market exclusivity (i.e. before the generic "substantially equivalent" are approved), just to cover the cost of introducing the original medication. Mind you that this type of revenue must derive solely from the sales of the drug in question, and does not include the company making any profit whatsoever.

Why is this so costly? To begin, only one in 1000 compounds that are tested in laboratories ever makes it to human testing. Once the FDA approves the IND (Figure 21-1), the drug must go through three phases of clinical trials:

1) <u>Phase 1</u>: Designed to establish the drug's safety profile by using it in 20-80 healthy volunteers.

2) <u>Phase 2</u>: Designed to assess the drug's effectiveness in 100-300 patient volunteers.

3) <u>Phase 3</u>: designed to determine effectiveness and adverse reactions in 1000-3000 actual patients.

Once these steps are completed, the company submits the NDA (this is typically about 100,000 pages) to the FDA for approval. This is the reason why it costs so much money to bring a brand-new medication to market. Curiously, one of the assumptions of the Hatch–Waxman Act was that the development of generic products prior to the expiration of patents would have minimal effects on brand-name medications. However, they never took into consideration how downgraded our system is and the effect of the control exerted by third-party payers (including Medicare and Medicaid) and their refusal to fund the use of brand-name medications once the "substantially equivalent" generic versions are available. This is a battle we fight on a daily basis, but it is one that we're losing due to acquiescence on the physicians' part in response to some of the hurdles we've already described or, more recently, to "bribes".[11] It is possible to see in this pattern of behavior how certain groups will believe what is convenient for them, in this case the entire sham of "bioequivalence", despite logic or reason. For example, pharmacists' profit margins are considerably higher when selling the generic version of any drug; a fact that is conveniently absent from the discussion of "conflicts of interest". Along the same lines of thought, another topic that has fascinated me is how groups of physicians completely obsessed with the concept of Evidence Based Medicine (EBM) as we discussed in Chapter 2, don't even give a second thought to the use of generic medications instead of the

---

[11] As this book is going to print, I have been informed that Blue Cross/Blue Shield of Alabama is about to start increasing reimbursement by 10% to physicians who prescribed generic medications for a majority of patients.

brand-name drugs tested in the published clinical trials (i.e. the actual "evidence") despite the differences pointed out. I have always wondered what would happen to the believed effectiveness of a certain medication based upon these clinical trials, if we were to factor in 20% less effectiveness due to the generic version's lower bioavailability (B in Figure 21-2). The result of all of this is a collusion that leads to treatment decisions being made on behalf of patients by individuals who bear no responsibility whatsoever relative to the clinical outcome. Downgraded enough for you?

Before concluding this chapter, I would like to share with you a thought that occurred to me while I was pondering about this whole topic. In our country, upon creating an original work of literature, music, art or computer software, the author is immediately endowed with what is known as *Copyright*. For example, the fact that you are reading this book means that I already have copyrights to it. I did not have to fill out a form, present any information anywhere, or even make a single phone call! More importantly, the copyrights of any author are protected for his entire lifespan, plus another 50 years. Even anonymous work is protected up to 100 years after its creation. On the other hand, to get a *patent* is a very convoluted process that requires for the individual or the organization to hire an expert attorney, and to spend a considerable amount of time and money seeing it to fruition. Patents are only granted by the federal government, and a last no more than 20 years, which is exactly the position of pharmaceutical companies when they introduce brand-new drugs. It seems to me, that there is a wide gap, an inappropriate disparity if you will, between these two processes. I suggest that one of the possible solutions to some of the problems of the cost of brand-name drugs, the fuel that incites the development of generic versions, is some type of reform of the current system by which it requires less government intervention and sanction. It is conceivable that, if a pharmaceutical company is not forced to recoup all the money invested in developing a drug within a very short and finite period of time, it will not find it necessary to price it at an exaggerated level. This way, it is also possible that the incentive to introduce generic versions of it will be minimized. A skeptic may ask: *"But, what about the risk of a monopoly?"* As it turns out, there is hardly any class of medications in which only one product is available! Thus, instead of promoting a brand name vs. generics competition, we would shift the paradigm to a brand name vs. brand name model. Just a thought...

In summary, generic medications have been allowed in our country as alternatives to brand name drugs after their patent has expired. Historically, the politics and legislation that have led to the current state of affairs have been somewhat convoluted and fraught with arbitrary decisions. Moreover, a close review of such history reveals the ever-present progressive practice of justifying change based on "crises" often fabricated from their interpretation of social incidents. According to the government, generic medications are "the same" that their brand-name counterparts, although their definition of "same" is more akin "equivalent", as determined by a shoddy process based on poor science and inappropriate use of statistics. The truth, particularly when we deal with medications that have a narrow therapeutic range, is that the use of generic versions of a drug may actually endanger the patient's life. Nevertheless, we are browbeaten daily by the government and its cronies to forcefully steer patients into taking generic drugs. The justification is... ... cost! What else? It is a sad day when the decision about what medication a patient is to take is compulsorily made by some flunky working for an insurance carrier; especially when he will not bear any responsibility for the outcome of the patient. That said, just like I mentioned in previous chapters, if the patients are unwilling to fight this fight by taking it as far as Congress if necessary, then they essentially are picking their own poison!

22

Paperwork

"The man whose life is devoted to paperwork has lost the initiative. He's dealing with things that are brought to his notice, having ceased to notice anything for himself."

C. Northcote Parkinson
British Naval Historian and Author
(1909 - 1993)

If my goal in life had been to fill out forms, I would have become a clerk, not a physician. However, after three decades of practice, I can honestly say that our current healthcare system views physicians largely as glorified secretaries. Not one week goes by in which one more form intended for us to complete does not appear in the hospital medical records. The problem has become so widespread and pervasive, that no one seems to find it astonishing, and evidently not as insulting as I do. I have always said that, just like police cars have the words *"To protect and to serve!"* printed on their side, perhaps physicians' vehicles should analogously display the statement *"To diagnose and to treat!"* since these two are our principal and only sworn duties. After all, nowhere in the

Hippocratic Oath does it say that we swear by Apollo to fill out all forms placed in front of us on behalf of the patient, regardless of how many there are or how stupid their construct is. Having said this, however, we must admit that the reason so many forms are incessantly being shoved in our path is because we have allowed it; we have even encouraged it by continuing to fill them out with very little resistance. Nevertheless, the situation is now beyond intolerable and I think it is only fair that I dedicate one chapter of the book to it, pointing out how this ever-increasing mound of paperwork contributes to the downgrading of our healthcare system.

Any discussion about paperwork relative to medical care must take into account the following dimensions: a) The patient's needs, b) The physician's duty, and c) The fairness of the clinical exchange. The first of these three dimensions is probably the easiest one to consider since I have already made my position clear elsewhere in the book: *"The patient gets what the patient needs"* (not what he "wants"). Let me emphasize again (as I covered in Chapter 18) that I consider giving into the patient "wants" a shift towards medicine *à la Carte* and the starting point of *the road to clinical serfdom*. In regards to the physician's duty, I have also categorically expressed how my view of this subject is bound by the primary components of the clinical encounter: *To diagnose and to treat!* Anything else is extra and, at least in principle, should be considered discretionary work on the part of the physician.

It is the last of the three dimensions where the argument about paperwork should be centered. Fairness as it relates to the clinical encounter is a concept that is not often discussed but one that becomes tangible in the context of how the two previous dimensions relate operationally. Once the physician fulfills his duty, and sees to the needs of the patient, he must complete the cycle of the encounter by documenting its particulars in as much detail as he can. This is fair and widely considered as the gold standard. Generally speaking, the one tool that is the direct work product of any clinical encounter, and therefore should be sufficient repository of relevant clinical information for any future query, is the *medical record* (Figure 22-1). Think about it; the medical record contains all the clinical data pertinent to the

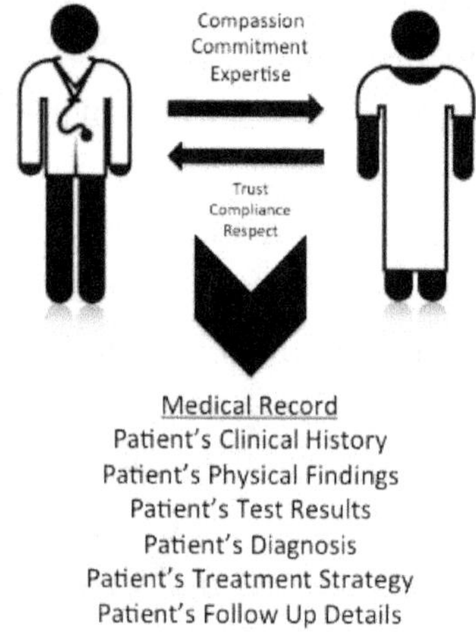

Figure 22-1
The Medical Record = The Work Product of the Encounter

patient and, as such, it should allow ANYONE to answer ANY question relative to the patient's medical status. As a matter of fact, my own medical records all incorporate discussions about the patient's condition at the time of the encounter, including commentaries about working capability or restrictions. Thus, why should I be coerced into completing forms by entering information I already recorded in my medical records? Why should I carry out duplicative and redundant work? I say *I should not have to do so!* I also say that anyone who wants the information already contained in my medical records to be neatly entered into his precious forms should compensate me for the extra time spent doing so! Otherwise, my message regarding the topic of paperwork is very clear: *All the patient's information should be in the medical record, and this should preclude the need for any forms to be completed!*

That said, I acknowledge that there are exceptions to my hardline argument. In some instances, the form being presented for our completion may actually be an utterly simple one that serves a specific purpose tethered to a medical opinion about a topic not commonly found in medical records. In instances such as this, I don't have a quarrel with the request and I am generally willing to oblige. This type of request includes a *de facto* necessary form, one for which there is no substitute and which serves a discrete and necessary role for the patient. For example, every state of the union in which I have worked has a form that allows a physician to certify that a patient is disabled and is entitled to get special license plates for his vehicle so he can park in disabled-only spaces. This type of form is simply irreplaceable and clearly needed. However, it is also one of the easiest forms to fill out since it relies solely on the opinion of the physician without asking for too many explanations. Its simplicity does not constitute a burden of any material magnitude and we gracefully complete it on demand. However, we are at a point in which we have included such form into our electronic medical records (EMR) and made its completion markedly easy.

Nonetheless, what happens when the form that is placed in front of us is convoluted, poorly designed, or asks for answers to stupid questions? Let me cite a simple and very common example: Many of the forms we are asked to complete require us to enter a blood pressure reading. Seriously? What purpose could a single discrete measurement of a continuous variable serve? Sorry, did I lose you? Let me explain! Blood pressure is a physiologic variable that exists all the time (i.e. continuously). It fluctuates throughout the day for a variety of reasons, some of which are simple biological rhythms. Thus, any single measurement (i.e. discrete) will NEVER reflect how the system that generates blood pressure operates *in toto*. No single measurement will ever be representative of the function itself and should not be used to make life-altering decisions. Now back to our discussion, to asking for a single blood pressure reading in a form is pointless, and utterly representative of the type of useless information that threatens to occupy our time unnecessarily. Moreover, since patients are examined multiple times over the course of their clinical care, which one of the blood pressure readings should we enter? Todays? Last visits? Anyway, you see my point... ...Senseless!

Hold on because it gets better! In addition to asking for ridiculous information, many forms require the physician to provide narrative explanations of an opinion issued (concurrently or previously) regarding the patient. For example, such requests commonly take the following format:

"Please list the objective findings that support your opinion:"

and/or

"Please list the results of the tests that support your conclusions:"

It is precisely this type of demand that validates my argument that this is nothing but wasteful and uncompensated re-work of information we have already recorded in the medical record. Hence, let's examine this issue from the perspective of queries such as those cited above, and the work product of the clinical encounter (Figure 25-1): The medical record comprises the clinical history of the patient (i.e. subjective), the physical examination (i.e. objective), the test results (i.e. ancillary data), the diagnoses (i.e. assessment), and treatment recommendations (i.e. plan). If you think about it, there's nothing else! There is no other *hidden* clinical information about the patient!

So, why is there such an insistence in forcing physicians to duplicate our work by simply copying the information that is in the medical record unto a form? The answer to this question is at the heart of the problem we are discussing. The simplest and most evident reason is that whoever is requesting completion of the form is either too lazy to review our medical records or not qualified to understand them. Believe me when I tell you that intellectual laziness and unqualified (i.e. cheap) labor have a way of finding each other, just so they can cozily hold hands as they torment the rest of us! Together they champion the endless utilization of forms to force others to do their job for them, and are pervasively present throughout the bureaucratic milieu of our system. However, and at the risk of sounding too paranoid, there certainly is another potential, more underhanded reason behind the paperwork tsunami we are currently weathering. I suggest that, when it comes to third party payers whose primary mission in life is to deny payment of claims made regardless of their legitimacy, forcing physicians to fill out forms creates one more hurdle that needs to be completed prior to disbursement of funds. It also provides them with a tool by which, should any portion of a form not be filled to their satisfaction (usually determined by a high school dropout clerk), payment can be denied until the form is "properly" completed. This game of reimbursement cat and mouse, which we largely addressed in Chapter 7, represents a major component of the indirect cost of healthcare in our country, and not a very broadcasted contributor to the increased cost of healthcare in general. Along these lines, there is all type of paperwork we come across on a daily basis. In the next few pages, I will discuss the most egregious but by no means the only ones.

One of the most condescending and downright insulting forms we are asked to complete is the infamous "Prior Authorization (PA)" form. If you are not familiar with it, let me introduce you to the process that is represents. It begins when we prescribe a medication that the patient's third party carrier (either an insurance company or Medicare/Medicaid) has chosen not to cover purely due to financial reasons, and under the incorrect assumption (fostered by their in-house pharmacists) that all drugs within a class (e.g. all beta blockers) are "therapeutically equivalent", and that generic medications are equivalent to the brand name drugs they intend to replace (you should be familiar with this topic after reading Chapter 21). In any case, as soon as the patient attempts to fill such a prescription, he is promptly notified that the third party payer is balking. But, he is also told that, should his physician complete a PA form and send it in they would be willing to reconsider their decision. How do you like them apples? The physician has to appeal for some pencil pusher to *authorize* his expert therapeutic decision! All those years of education, and all those licenses and board certifications undermined by bureaucrats working at a half-ass educational level!

What is the immediate result? An annoyed patient demanding that we fill one this PA forms so he can get his medication! What information is required in the PA form? We already covered this; the same that is already in the medical record! Despite this fact, the third party payer will not accept anything but their form, undoubtedly for the reasons we listed above. At this time, pushed into a corner by the conjoined demands of patient and payer, physicians traditionally have followed one of several alternative courses of action:

1) Acquiesce and complete the form. Which does not guarantee that the patient will get the medication prescribed, as you will see below.

2) Acquiesce and change the prescription for one of their recommended "therapeutic equivalents". Which will end the standoff by an admission on the part of the physician that his original decision was not necessarily correct.

3) Appeal the decision and request to speak with one of their clinical decision-makers (i.e. a physician or pharmacist reviewer). Which typically leads to painful conversations with ignoramuses.

As you can easily see, the common denominator of all three choices is additional time and effort expenditure on the part of the physician. Bravo! They have managed to take a menial clerical process and converted it into an all around duplicative, redundant and confrontational exercise right on the physician's face! Welcome to my world!

Let's expand on each of the alternatives facing the physician whenever a PA form is requested of him, particularly because similar courses of action are generally comparable for nearly any other form. Imagine he goes ahead and completes the PA form, signs it, and sends it in. Note that, by proceeding in this course of action, the physician is asserting that in his expert opinion the medication in question is the best choice for the patient's treatment. The most common response this action gets is that, according to the carrier's rules, the medication requested will not be covered unless the patient has "failed" one of their suggested therapeutic equivalents. Now, let's think about this for a moment. The argument we made in Chapter 21 about generic drugs applies perfectly in this situation. If the proposed therapeutic equivalent is used to lower cholesterol, its so-called "failure" may be uncovered the next time blood work is carried out. However, if the purpose of the therapeutic equivalent is to prevent stroke, do we really want the patient to "fail"? Naturally, this asinine response on the part of the carrier is always accompanied with the option to appeal the decision (identical to number 3 above). Other times, less commonly, sending a completed PA form leads to a phone call by one of the carrier's reviewers (i.e. the ignoramuses I mentioned earlier) with the consequent interaction being similar to that described in the paragraphs below. On a somewhat humorous personal note, I have always thought that the verbal counterpart of filling out the PA form would sound something like *"I really, really meant to prescribe this medication!"* It is equivalent to begging for our expert opinion to be taken into consideration. Not very dignified if you ask me!

Now, let's say the physician takes the second path and changes the prescription to one of the suggested therapeutic equivalents. In the first place, he is admitting that there is really no difference between the drug he originally prescribed and the alternative. So, he has avoided wasting time completing the PA form, but he still has to do re-work by writing a new prescription. Candidly, physicians have been beaten so much over this topic through the years, that this is the most common course of action. However, I have several questions relevant to this topic before I move on: If the physician changes the prescription to the suggested alternative, and the patient "fails" therapy and gets hurt, is he liable? Is the carrier ever liable? Is anyone liable for this aspect of medical care? Who is responsible for the "failed" outcome? In my view, answers to these questions are of enormous importance and yet, it is not a subject openly discussed. As you may realize by now, I have a real problem with individuals (e.g. pharmacists) and organizations (e.g. insurance carriers) making decisions about patients' care but bearing no responsibility of its consequences. Keep reading because it gets better...

The third pathway leads to one of the most painful exercises in futility I have ever encountered. Typically, the carrier provides us with the telephone number of a reviewer physician in their employment, and asks us to call and request "authorization" for the original prescription. Mind you, that the reviewer may be someone no longer in practice, or in practice in a totally different specialty. The point is that the reviewer's questions are usually obtuse and pointless. In fact, it is the physician who has the upper hand and not uncommonly can get the prescription authorized, obviously by having to drop everything else he is doing to devote time and effort to this phone call. Personally, I refuse to have to explain myself to clerical or suboptimal clinical personnel. Furthermore, I also think that it is the patient who should be fighting his carrier and not the physician. The patient is the carrier's client, the one that in some way has paid the premiums, and the one being shortchanged. Given the opportunity, I usually give the reviewer's number to the patient and have him call directly, having instructed them to ask the following questions: *"Can you explain how can you decide to deny authorization for my prescription without ever having seen me?" "Can you describe your experience in treating conditions similar to mine?" "If my prescription is denied, will you be responsible for any harm that comes to me?"* The authorization is almost immediate!

Another paperwork nemesis is the Family Medical Leave Act (FMLA) form. The FMLA is a federal law signed by President Bill Clinton in 1993, to assured that employers would provide family and medical unpaid leave to employees under qualified circumstances. Once again, the government acted on what at first seems to be a good idea, without a thoughtful assessment of the potential unintended consequences derived from it. Now, I am not even going to address the so-called qualified reasons for coverage under this law since they are not relevant to our present discussion. However, I would like to contrast the original language of the law (Figure 22-2), with the paperwork that we are expected to take on as a result of its implementation.

Please examine figure 22-2 carefully. It is the actual language of the FMLA. I dare you to find anywhere in the statutes where it says that physicians must fill out any forms! What? Not there? Imagine that! The truth is that the FMLA form in question, also known as the WH-380-E form, is an afterthought of the law itself. A tool someone created for his own benefit, in order to force people to provide him with information in a neatly organized way that he could digest. I thought of including WH-380-E as an appendix but it is very easy to find a copy in the Internet. I encourage you to do so. It encompasses four pages. The employer has about one-third of a page to fill out. The employee has one line signature. The physician (excuse me, the "healthcare provider") has three and a half pages of questions and narrative. The sad thing is that the information required to complete WH-380-E is already in the medical record and, therefore, completing it is duplicative and redundant. In my view, all the FMLA literally requires is for the physician to provide "certification" of the

SEC. 103. CERTIFICATION.

(a) IN GENERAL.--An employer may require that a request for leave... ...be supported by a certification issued by the health care provider of the eligible employee or of the [family member] as appropriate. The employee shall provide, in a timely manner, a copy of such certification to the employer.

(b) SUFFICIENT CERTIFICATION.--Certification provided under subsection (a) shall be sufficient if it states

(1) the date on which the serious health condition commenced;

(2) the probable duration of the condition;

(3) the appropriate medical facts within the knowledge of the health care provider regarding the condition;

(4) ... ...[Need statements depending on reason for certification]

Figure 22-2
Actual Text of the FMLA (See Text for Explanation)

items listed. Since the bulk of these items are part of the medical record, I insist that the latter should suffice. Since there is also an element of opinion that may not be typically part of the medical record, a simple cover form in which these are addressed should also suffice. This is what I have implemented in our practice using output from our EMR, very successfully I may add. It passes the litmus test of fairness for the medical encounter since it involves minimal extra expenditure of time and effort, and hardly any duplication or redundant work. Does this approach work all the time? Not at all! As I mentioned earlier, the combination of intellectual laziness and unqualified labor rears its ugly head often enough to cause trouble by virtue of certain organization (typically government agencies) demanding that we complete WH-380-E, and refusing to accept our method of providing certification as the law prescribes. In these cases, I usually advise the patients to discuss the matter with their attorney or their congressman. Ah! The congressman! A very underutilized resource in this type of bureaucratic altercation! I will expand on this topic in the next few pages.

Another set of forms that clutter our daily practice are those that relate to the application of therapy (i.e. physical, occupational, speech) to patients. In my view, these forms represent one of the most corrupt and wasteful processes of medical care. Here is how it works: Let's say we order physical therapy for a patient with a lumbar disc herniation and back pain. We send the orders, the patient goes to a local therapy center, and then the therapist writes up a treatment plan and sends it for our signature. Why? Because the rules are that he will not be able to get paid unless we sign off and approve the plan. Mind you that I now have to spend more of my time reviewing the paperwork, signing it and sending it back. At least in this case I should be elated that Medicare allows payment of $48.50 for my effort. Wow! I guess now I can have that operation... So, instead of treating the therapists like professionals (which is what they want anyway) and auditing them directly, they stick the physician in the middle as the arbiter of a murky process. One that has become increasingly obtrusive, to the point that its latest addition is... ...Guess what? One more form called the *"Face-to-Face Documentation Form"*. Seriously? By now you should have guessed what my next objection is going to be: Isn't the encounter already recorded in the medical record a face-to-face meeting?

So far, we have been discussing paperwork in the ambulatory care setting, but what about the forms inside the hospital charts? These are also a major hindrance and generally relate to quality indicators or regulations issued by the government or its surrogates [e.g. The Joint Commission (TJC)]. At the time of this writing, the most notorious include: the patient restraint form, the deep venous thrombosis (DVT) prophylaxis form, and the Medicare Core Measures form. Their common denominator includes the fact that they are unnecessary, do not help patients in any way, and occupy our time. In addition, they come with a cadre of minions who are bound and determined to force us to fill out these forms, irrespective of what other patient-related activity this hampers. I think I have covered *ad nauseam* my objections to all the regulations and protocols in previous chapters. The forms I am now referring to are simply the tools that detail these processes so the hospital can document its compliance with the mandates. Let me share an anecdote that represents an example of their unreasonableness: One of my colleagues tells about how irritated he became when one of the hospital quality watchdogs insisted that he completed the DVT prophylaxis form in the chart of a stroke patient who was ambulatory! Let me explain some more: The prophylaxis (i.e. prevention) of DVT is one of the core measures enforced by TJC in the context of stroke care. It relates to the use of processes to prevent the formation of blood clots in the calf veins of patients who cannot move their legs. However, by definition, a patient who is walking about does not need any of such measures, a fact in evidence by reading the hospital chart! Despite this, the hospital minion insisted that the physician completed the form! This is what we have to endure on a daily basis: a downgraded system in which the outcome of the patient care does not matter... *...so long as all forms are properly completed!*

So, is there a solution? I say there is! It consists of a two-step answer to the queries that forms represent. First, widespread physician refusal to complete unnecessary forms, with automatic referral to the medical record as the work product of the clinical encounter; let them read the answers in the chart and, if they do not understand the chart, let them go and get an education! Second, have patients take responsibility for this fight! It is, after all, their problem and they should be "empowered" (using the current fashionable term) to address it. Also, advise them to discuss the matter with their congressman; I am firmly convinced that if our congressmen were to receive 100-200 letters per day denouncing this (or any other healthcare problem), written by registered voters, stupid situations such as this would be fixed within weeks.

In summary, paperwork has become one of the most ubiquitous hurdles to the practice of medicine. The number of forms we are constantly asked to complete, typically spending our time and effort without any compensation, grows almost exponentially and in parallel with the expansion of regulatory mandates. The cultural changes that underlie this process center on the notion that the paperwork is more important than the work itself! In general, the information required in these forms is redundant from that already contained in the medical record; the work product of the clinical process. Therefore, it is simply unreasonable to continue to ask physicians to carry out duplicative work, and it is senseless for us to comply with a process that is beyond our sworn duty. As such, patients need to understand that anything asked beyond our scope of practice cannot become our added responsibility, and that it is up to them to squash unreasonable requests made by the government or by insurance carriers. To this end, they should always consider involving their congressmen to the extent that they provide the leverage necessary to change what is clearly a downgrading aberration of the current system.

23

Patient Privacy

"The privacy and dignity of our citizens are being whittled away by sometimes imperceptible steps. Taken individually, each step may be of little consequence. But when viewed as a whole, there begins to emerge a society quite unlike any we have seen - - a society in which government may intrude into the secret regions of a person's life."

William O. Douglas
Associate Justice of the U.S. Supreme Court
(1898 - 1980)

As far back as I can remember, the privacy of patients' medical information has been an explicit concern for all of us involved in the practice of medicine. However, leave it to the government to take action with the excuse of "protecting the public interest" to give the entire concept of medical information privacy a double dose of anabolic steroids and, as a result, creating an Orwellian electronic infrastructure worthy of any notion one may have about "Big Brother". Such an arrangement finds its legal footing in the Health Insurance Portability and Accountability Act (HIPAA).

In 1996, then U.S. President Bill Clinton took time from his busy progressive agenda to sign the HIPAA. This piece of legislation, sponsored by a republican congresswoman from Kansas, consisted of two distinct parts. Title I was concerned with the ability of individuals to keep their health insurance coverage when they change or lose their jobs. Title II, also known as the Administrative Simplification (AS) provisions was more concerned with the establishment of standards for electronic medical transactions, the creation of national identifiers and, get this... the implementation of security and privacy measures relative to medical information of patients. I don't know about you, but I began to worry the moment I was informed that a government-run program was going to bring *administrative simplification!* Call me crazy but when is the last time our federal government did anything that simplifies our lives? You can go ahead and write me if you ever find an answer to this question!

In any case, it is precisely these AS provisions that are the subject of our discussion in this chapter. However, before we embark on our journey of what's private and how the government is going to help us keep it so, let me clarify my intent to go over Title I of HIPAA in my final conclusions of the book since I consider it redundant to aspects of the Affordability Care Act (ACA) (i.e. Obamacare). To provide you with an overview, Title II of HIPAA defines policies, procedures and guidelines for maintaining the privacy and security of patient medical information, outlines offenses relative to healthcare, specifies penalties for these violations, and creates several programs to control fraud and abuse within the healthcare system. In general, all of these aspects of Title II have not been as popularized as the AS provisions.

The latter, as promulgated by the Department of Health and Human Services (DHHS), include five distinct rules:

1) The Privacy Rule. This is precisely the subject of our discussion in this book chapter. The remaining rules, although also interesting topics of discussion, are somewhat subordinate to the Privacy Rule. Having become effective in April of 2003 (with a few exceptions), it regulates the use and disclosure of Protected Health Information (PHI) by the so-called "covered entities" and their "business associates". The former include essentially everyone involved in medical care, from the bedside (e.g. physicians and nurses) through the compensation process (e.g. clearinghouses and payers). The latter Refers to any independent contractor of the covered entities. By PHI, this law interprets any part of an individual's medical record or payment history. Finally, it stipulates standards by which covered entities must provide PHI to individual patients upon request, and disclose them where prescribed by law (e.g. child abuse).

2) The Transactions and Code Sets Rule. Since HIPAA was supposed to make our healthcare system more efficient (Yes! You read correctly...), it was used to modify the Social Security Act (SSA) that requires all health plans to engage in healthcare transactions in a standardized way. This is known as the Electronic Data Interchange (EDI), and due to significant confusion and difficulty in its implementation (Imagine that!), it only became effective in October of 2004. In fact, after July of 2005, most covered entities were required to file electronic claims using the HIPAA standards if they wanted to get reimbursed! Again, at the risk of sounding skeptical, it

seems to me that this is just another form of government control of how the processes operate. Furthermore, I cannot help but think, *"He who makes the rules, also makes the traps!"* The simple fact that it is the government that has set the standards that govern how electronic medical data are to be maintained and transmitted, should cast a shadow of doubt about real privacy of any of this information.

3) The Security Rule. This provision, with effect on April of 2003, is intended to complement the Privacy Rule. It specifies three types of security safeguards required for compliance pertinent to Electronic Protected Health Information (EPHI): a) Administrative, b) Physical, and c) Technical. As you can imagine, each of these three includes a set of standards that span all the way from policies and procedures, all the way to hardware and software specifications that must be effected by they covered entity in order to be compliant. Let me point out again that these rules were supposed to provide administrative simplification.

4) The Unique Identifiers Rule. This provision requires all covered entities to use only the National Provider Identifier (NPI) number to recognize covered healthcare providers in any of the standard transactions described. This rule became effective in May of 2007. The NPI replaces all other identifiers used by either the government or private insurance carriers, but it does not replace the Drug Enforcement Administration (DEA) number, state license number, or tax identification number. Well, it feels like we have been "tagged", and I am simply surprised that they have not required us to

have the NPI number tattooed in our forearm. Too harsh? Keep reading...

5) <u>The Enforcement Rule</u>. This one became effective in March of 2006, and includes civil money penalties for violating HIPAA rules. It also establishes the format for investigations and hearings pertinent to HIPAA violations.

Now that we have walked you through the highlights of the AS provisions, let us discuss further how this whole cadre of new regulations impacts your privacy, and our way of delivering care. Before I dwell into these two important topics, let me also point out that, within the scope of HIPAA, there are special considerations for confidentiality required from covered entities involved in federally funded drug or alcohol rehabilitation services. These exist in the context of the Comprehensive Alcohol Abuse and Alcoholism Prevention, Treatment and Rehabilitation Act of 1970, as well as the Drug Abuse Office and Treatment Act of 1972. I bring this up because when we start looking at solutions for the future of medical care, I submit that we will have to come to grips with the reality of choosing what roles do alcohol and drug abuse programs play within the scope of medical practice. For example, if we embrace the idea that both alcoholism and drug abuse are medical conditions, no different from hypertension or diabetes in this sense, and "nothing to be ashamed of", then why would they need special confidentiality provisions? Conversely, if they are simply the result of improper social choices, why should they be considered part of medical care at all?

So, how did we get to this point in our quest for privacy? Traditionally, patient's confidentiality has been a major concern in medical practice. Even the Hippocratic Oath contained a reference to this topic: *"What I may see or hear in the course of the treatment or even outside of the treatment in regard to the life of men, which on no account one must spread abroad, I will keep to myself..."* Hence, as far back as I can remember, we have considered the information provided by the patient or pertinent to him, sacred and strictly confidential. That said, we have always had that attitude and discretionary judgment that relates to specific scenarios in which sharing certain patient care information with others was necessary. For example, in discussing the case with a colleague while we ask for advice (i.e. second opinion), or discussing aspects of the care of a comatose patient who has no family with a close friend that may help in our decision about the best way to help the patient. Typically, these situations have resulted in no harm to anyone and arguably have contributed to the care the patient. So, it begs the question, why did we need a massive government intervention to "improve" how patients' information is maintained private and confidential? Moreover, why is our industry singled out when in fact private and confidential information shared with attorneys, accountants, or bankers is no less of potential harm to individuals if "shared" inappropriately? Interestingly, my review of the subject left me somewhat unsatisfied due to the lack of objective evidence that, in my view, would justify the creation of HIPAA. The most widely cited reason behind it is the need to *"improve the efficiency and effectiveness of the health care system by standardizing the electronic exchange of administrative and financial data."* In fact, there are those who think that the government *"came to the rescue only because the healthcare industry failed to work toward this goal."* Interestingly, however, statements such as this are followed by an argument that includes the government's belief that, by encouraging electronic transactions, the cost of healthcare would decrease significantly and efficiencies would be gained. Now, let's not forget that this is the same government that believes that selectively giving money to companies such as Solyndra is the way to grow a sector of the energy production market! Along the same lines, it is also possible to find statements addressing the concerns of legislators that advance in electronic technology would place an increased risk to the patient's privacy. Wait a minute! I thought we were talking about improving efficiency and effectiveness? Well, as it often happens with government work, they began with an idea and a purpose, and started to pile more things onto them. Should there have been a concern about patient's confidentiality? Reports of pharmacies legally selling individual prescription records the pharmaceutical companies, or mailing list brokers selling the names of patients with one or another condition abound. Furthermore, there have been clearly illegal breaches of confidentiality such as a public health worker in Florida who leaked the names of thousands of HIV patients to newspapers. Thus, the answer to the aforementioned question is yes! But I submit but there probably were already laws in the books that would have allowed these incidents to be properly addressed. This brings us to the theme that would be important as we wind down the book and head towards finding a potential solution to our downgraded healthcare system: *More laws, and certainly a bigger government, are definitely not the answer!*

The negative impact of the improper dissemination of medical information is not something to be taken lightly. That said, we have to critically analyze whether introducing all of these standards has actually improved our situation or just simply has created more energy expenditure. In the words of the late coach John Wooden: *"Never mistake activity for achievement!"* The first argument about the potential benefit of the Privacy Rule is that it sets the national standards for handling medical information. On the surface, this seems like a good deal! Who would not want homogeneity in how the information is acquired, stored, analyzed, and transmitted between two or more covered entities? However, between 2006 and 2007, well after these regulations had been required, a recent study reported 1.5 million instances of data breaches in hospitals; without including order types of covered entities. It is impossible to know how this figure compares with breaches of confidentiality prior to the introduction of HIPPA regulations. However, I argue that despite all the money and time that have been spent trying to fix this problem, it remains alive and well! Should this be surprising? In my view, the dishonesty or the carelessness that are at the root of breaches of patient confidentiality will continue to exist despite any changes we make in the system because both are human conditions. Furthermore, experts in data security suggest that HIPAA fails to adequately protect patient data due to its lack of oversight, guidance and enforcement. They point out that the organizations being trusted to protect medical data are not in the data protection business, and suggest that a better model may perhaps be involving the Data Security Standard (DSS) being used by the credit card industry. Finally, there are those who think that HIPAA's Privacy Rule is actually nothing more than a disclosure regulation; and that it doesn't protect privacy of patients since it allows easy dissemination without audit trails for most disclosures. This is an interesting point of view; one that will lead us to address potential problems regarding HIPAA and the use of confidential patient information.

I think it is important that, before we continue our discussion, we consider the fact that in providing this gargantuan legislation, the government once again has justified it as looking to protect the patients' "Right to Privacy". Proof of this is the fact that they have appointed the Office of Civil Rights (OCR) of the DHHS as the enforcer of the Privacy Rule. Let's see how that is working out under HIPAA:

1) The patient's consent is not required when medical information is disclosed relative to treatment, payment or healthcare operations.

2) The patient's past medical information may become available despite the fact that he may think it would never come up.

3) The patient's medical information can be used for marketing without explicit authorization.

4) The patient has no right to sue under HIPAA for violations.

5) The patient's medical information can be disclosed to business associates of a covered entity without knowledge or consent.

A close look at these shortcomings of HIPAA clearly establishes the fact that, just as it has happened in many other occasions, the real intent is for the government to protect its right to manage medical information pertinent to our population. This is a very important concept; at the heart of the debate between freedom of the individual and the rights of the collective. Make no mistake; granting the government the right to control medical information is an important step towards total government oversight of the medical treatment cycle, including decisions about who gets what care and who doesn't. I don't know about you, but it sounds a lot like rationing to me!

There are other aspects of HIPPA that allegedly benefit patients. For example, the patient has the right to access his own medical records. However, in reading this I felt like we had just discovered warm water! When I was a little boy, growing up in Venezuela, the pediatrician all of the children in our family used to go to, never kept office medical records. Remember, this is well before we had computers or even pocket calculators! His system was to make entries about each visit in a binder that he would promptly returned to the child's mother for safekeeping. This meant that she had access to the information (provided she could understand his handwriting), and this would be available in case the family was to travel taking the child somewhere else. I always found this to be a very interesting and effective system. Against this backdrop, throughout my career, I have always taken the position that any of my patients is granted immediate access to his medical records upon request. After all, it is their information and I do not need some government official to tell me that. In fact, I still offer my patients the opportunity to get all of their existing medical records from our office if they just bring with them a computer thumb drive that we can copy them onto. That way, if they travel someplace else, it would be very easy for some other covered entity to view the information in their Portable Document Format (PDF) files.

So, what happens when HIPAA rules are not followed? As we noted earlier, the OCR is charged with enforcing the Privacy Rule in the midst of enforcing all other civil rights laws. Its specific directives are to promote voluntary compliance, investigate and resolve complaints, and determine exceptions. The first of his three is laughable because it pretends that covered entities are willing to comply voluntarily with what is clearly a compulsory process. It is nothing more than the government "sugarcoating" the entire endeavor. I have yet to find anyone who is complying with any of these regulatory requirements voluntarily. I submit that everyone does it for fear of the penalties imposed for not acquiescing. Along this line, any person or organization may file a HIPAA violation complaint with OCR, and individuals may also file complaints directly with covered entities. To reiterate, however, the patient has no right to a claim for a HIPAA violation; only the DHHS or the Department of Justice (DOJ) can pursue such course. The penalties for violating HIPAA regulations can be civil or criminal. The former include $100 per violation and are capped at $25,000 for each calendar year, but the latter can go as high as $250,000 and 10 years of imprisonment, and are enforced by the DOJ.

Let's turn our attention to the consequences of HIPAA on medical practice and clinical research. In the first place, the uncertainty secondary to the complexity of HIPAA, combined with the fear of the potential penalties for violations has led to many covered entities to withhold information from entities with the right to have it. Also, in order to become compliant, covered entities have been forced to spend considerable amount of money in developing and revamping systems, while in fact they have seen their amount of paperwork and staff time necessary for this process, increase. At a time when reimbursement for medical services continues to decline, the formula resulting from this is an assault on the solvency of any of these organizations. Finally, there has been significant amount of financial and energy expenditure in the education and training of providers in order to ensure they comply with these regulations. Relative to research activities, the HIPPA regulations have clearly affected and changed the ability to perform retrospective, chart-based, studies. Moreover, it has become increasingly difficult to prospectively evaluate patients by contacting them for follow-up. There have been reports of substantial drops in research patients' follow-up from major universities and there's a distinct feeling among the research community that HIPAA has had a widespread negative effect on the cost and quality of medical research.

And then, just when we thought it was safe to go back in the water, our paternalistic government gave us the Health Information Technology for Economic and Clinical Health Act (HITECH) as part of the American Recovery and Reinvestment Act (ARRA) of 2009 (i.e. the stimulus bill). This set of regulations were justified by the idea that it was not sufficient for covered entities to adopt Electronic Medical Records (EMR),[12] but to also to embrace their *"Meaningful Use"* (MU). This is a term that I have introduced before in several chapters and that I would like to expand upon some more at this time. The main components of MU are:

1) <u>The use of a certified EMR in a meaningful manner</u>.

---

[12] The government uses the term Electronic Health Records, or EHR, but I am unwilling to give up EMR for reasons that should be clear by now

2) <u>The use of certified EMR technology for electronic information exchange to improve quality</u>.

3) <u>The use of certified EMR technology to submit clinical quality and other measures</u>.

In other words, the government insists that providers demonstrate that they are using EMR technology in ways that can be measured. Again, besides being a government control scheme since some of the data required for MU has nothing to do with good clinical outcomes, they have added a bribery component by which providers who comply with these requirements can earn up to $63,750 over six years from 2011. This amounts to a little more than $10,000 pear year and does not take into consideration the money that each provider would be required to spend to achieve such a payment. More importantly, physicians who do not adopt EMR by 2015 will be penalized 1% of Medicare payments, increasing to 3% over three years. As if our services are not already discounted enough! Please do not let it escape from your attention that it is the government that certifies EMR technology and therefore dictates the MU information that must be acquired and how is acquired. It then turns around, and exercises financial pressures to compel covered entities to follow the MU path that has been laid in front of them. You are now looking at the full operational circle of government control of medical information!

I cannot finish the chapter without at least saying some words about EMR. This is one of the best ideas with the worst possible executions I have ever seen! I have been a proponent of EMR for many years. In fact, having done programming and database design in the past, as early as 1999 we had implemented a homegrown version of a simple

EMR in our service at UAB (both inpatient and outpatient). Once I stepped outside and started to use different commercial versions of EMR, I have had every conceivable trouble with them; and this was before MU was even in the radar screen! From the design point of view, an EMR has four components, each vulnerable to the effect of ignoramuses being involved in the construction process. The effect of flawed EMR designs on the practice of medicine has been witnessed by physician after physician who has been forced to use them. It would not be proper for me to touch on this point without a least sharing my two-cents worth of what I have learned about the four components of EMR:

1) Data Input. Clinically important data must be entered into the record of every patient, together with demographic information (i.e. patient identifiers), and billing information. Technology has advanced to the point where it is possible to enter the information by multiple means. For example, in our clinic it can be keyed into computers, scanned in, electronically uploaded, or dictated via voice recognition software. The point is, however, that different members of the staff can take advantage of the various methods for data entry depending upon what their roles are. One of the most important problems we have had is the insistence of EMR vendors in forcing physicians to enter their part of the clinical record by means that many find impractical, such as clicking on a tablet or using a keyboard. A great deal of the problem is the conflict between having an EMR which is robust for clinical documentation, or one whose strength is acquiring compliance information necessary for optimal billing and reimbursement; the latter is also known as a Practice Management Software. In the majority of cases, at least

until recently, most vendors could only provide excellence in one of these two domains, but not both.

2) Relational Database. The robustness of a good EMR is directly related to how well designed the background relational database is. Unfortunately, many of their programming geniuses behind the existing EMR products, know very little about database design, and I have found countless egregious errors in most of the products I have used. In fact, even with those that I have used the longest, I have had to spend a considerable amount of my time trying to reconcile the flow of information so it meets my clinical needs, because the database is poorly designed. The future for this aspect of EMR is now under the control of the government since they will dictate what data are going to be considered within MU! God help us all!

3) Work Product Output. In the last chapter, I repeatedly noted how the work product of the clinical encounter is the medical record of the patient. Therefore, for it to be "meaningful", it has to be of clinical value to anyone else that reads it. However, for all the grandiose production of HITECH, the overwhelming majority of the clinical notes describing the encounter between the patient and the physician, and produced by EMRs across the country have almost no clinical meaning! Believe me, I am not making this up! Moreover, the majority of seasoned clinicians agree with me. The typical output note from an EMR-recorded encounter reads like machine language. It contains seven or eight pages of compliance-related data that allows the physician to get reimbursed but that do nothing to improve clinical communication or patient

outcome. It is in this domain that I have spent hundreds of hours to tweak the output of my EMR until I have been satisfied that it reads as a traditional clinical note of two pages. Sure, we collect all the compliance and MU data required but, since such information is only important to the government, I don't have to put it in my daily notes even though we keep it safe and tight within our computers as the law prescribes!

4) Connectivity. I think this is what provided the government with the justification to intervene and create the chaos they have given us. Because of the differences in database design between the numerous EMR vendors, it was impossible to take information from one EMR and transmitted to another one (i.e. the data fields did not match). I submit, however, that the government has created a monstrosity of a system when all we needed was a homogeneous database design. Ah! And let's not forget that the EMR needs to connect to the clearinghouses that will assure reimbursement, which in turn have their own software requirements. From this point of view, we could stand tall and say, *"We asked for it!"*

Let me emphasize that, at its core, MU requires providers to transmit to the government what it considers quality indicators. How this information will be used, other than to withhold payment for covered entities that "do not meet the standard" is now uncertain.

In summary, patient privacy and confidentiality have been of paramount importance to physicians since the beginning of time. Government intervention by means of complex and convoluted legislation, introduced with the excuse that it is necessary to "protect the patient's privacy" has added a number of hurdles to the practice of medicine. Conversely, its benefit in terms of securing privacy or improving the quality of the clinical exchange is, at best, suspect. More importantly, at a time when the government insists that it is protecting the patients' rights pertinent to the confidentiality of medical information, it is requiring an increasingly large number of data points to be transmitted for centralized assessment of quality of care. It is difficult to understand how, on one hand, most of us feel that we have a gun pointed to our head with a demand to protect patient information, while on the other, the government continues to collect data that could be used in one of many ways to control the access to medical care. Although I still think EMR is a good idea, I can attest that its execution has been incredibly clumsy and counterproductive. If you are inclined to disagree with me about this point, I invite you to try to understand the clinical note produced by your physician after your last clinic visit. After all, you are entitled to look at it!

Final Remarks & Outlook

"All that is necessary for the forces of evil to win in the world is for enough good men to do nothing"

Edmund Burke
Irish Statesman, Author, Political Theorist and Philosopher
(1729 - 1797)

So, how do we fix the system without the necessity for a nuclear explosion that would level the field and force us to start from scratch? I have been wondering the same thing while I wrote page after page of this book. After all, we have taken a simple paradigm [Figure A (Reproduced from Figure 1-1)], and converted it into a convoluted, inefficient, bureaucratic, and ineffective system (Figure B). I have also wondered if in fact the situation is hopeless or not. I really do not know the answer to the last question, especially the day I am writing these passages when, in an astonishing decision, the Supreme Court of the United States (SCOTUS) upheld the constitutionality of the Affordable Care Act (ACA) (i.e. Obamacare) individual mandate. However, I know this: *If we stand idle and do nothing, the future will only bring about the reign of mediocrity in medicine for generations to come.*

In my view, the only solution that has any hope of reversing the current downgrading of American healthcare must be based on two distinct components: One *philosophical* and one *practical*. The *philosophical* component requires the establishment of a rational framework based upon a return to the fundamental core values of the practice of medicine (Figure A). It is only from this position that we will be able to design a practical strategy for implementing sensible and meaningful changes. Such a strategy, the *practical* component, must then be grounded on a solid concept: *The Free Market!* In the next pages, I would like to discuss the two

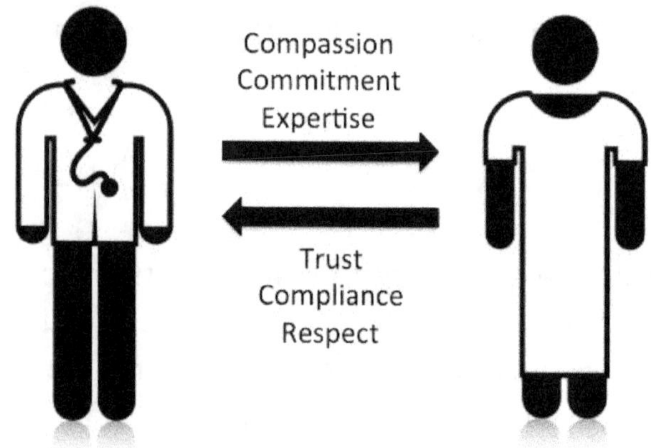

Figure A (Reproduced from Figure 1-1)
The Fundamental Physician-Patient Relationship

components of the solution I propose, expanding both of them in the context of the decisions that previously have gotten us to where we presently are. I would also like to familiarize the reader with the realization that many of the arguments used to get our system to the deplorable state in which it currently is, are the half-truths, uncritical concepts, and fabrications needed in order to advance a specific political progressive agenda.

In considering the *philosophical component* of our solution, we first must ponder what are the fundamental core values of medical practice that could provide the rationality that we need. Such a reflective exercise can only have one logical outcome: Once again we are compelled to embrace the central relationship between a physician and a patient (Figure A) as the pillar of the system, and to move back to the operating concept of *"Medical Care"* rather than the politically correct yet artificial one of "Healthcare". These two

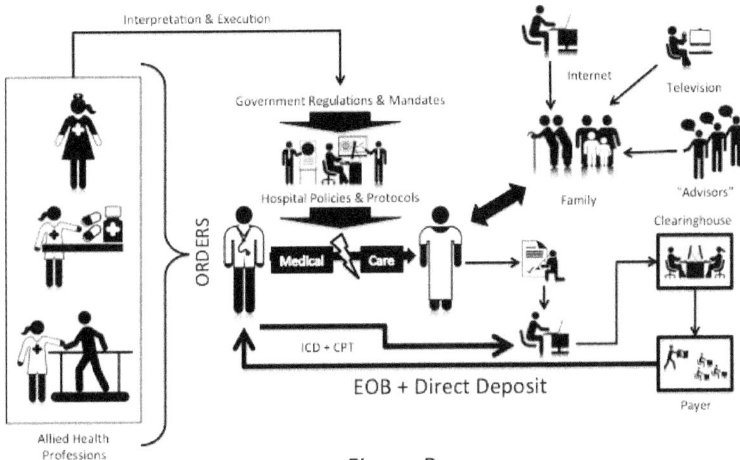

Figure B
The Current Paradigm of Medical Care (i.e. "Healthcare")

seemingly simple steps may be easier said than done, but we have got to start somewhere. Let's discuss each of them, and explain their potential implications.

I submit that nothing else will matter unless we first recognize the paramount importance of the relationship between the patient and his physician; unless we strengthen it, develop it, nurture it, allow it to mature, and make it the centerpiece of anything related to the delivery of medical care. Unlike the current obsession with making medical care "patient-centered", I contend that we are missing the mark by not grasping the true role of the physician-patient relationship as the real focus of any meaningful medical care strategy. In fact, unless we acknowledge the critical duality of this relationship, comparable only to marriage or to a very close partnership, we will fail miserably in driving the changes that will be needed in order to restore medical care to its rightful path. As I have pointed elsewhere in the book, "centering" care on the patient is comparable to founding the success of any marriage on the happiness of only one of the two spouses! Does that sound reasonable? Not even close! I say let's concentrate in fostering and encouraging both parties to live up to their end of the medical contract (Figure A) so there is an ongoing balance in their relationship, and so they both benefit from it. In pursuing this model, we would be bound to consider both parties as equal and, in doing so we would empower them as a complementary unit. This would then translate in every other aspect of the system, and every other individual who thinks of himself as a "stakeholder", becoming subordinate to this fundamental *unit of care*. It would also subordinate every activity related to medical care to the decisions made by the patient and the physician *together*. Finally, promoting such a dual partnership model would eradicate once and for all the concept of "firing" a physician, or a patient for that matter. As equals, either party could only "separate" from the other should irreconcilable differences arise, without having a position of subservience or undue supremacy. I submit that this is a more productive, fair and efficient model. So, you may ask, *"What role would families play in this model?"* My answer is simple: supplementary and adjuvant! Again, as I have expressed elsewhere in the book, unless the patient is a minor, or mentally incompetent in some way, I find the current behavior of many families often disrespectful (to both the patient and the physician), usurpative, and self-centered.

Continuing our discussion of the *philosophical component* of our solution, let's consider the importance of switching back to "Medical Care" from "Healthcare". Although at first this may seem just a matter of semantics, I submit that it represents the keystone of any future practical improvement of our system. Let me reiterate what I have already expressed elsewhere in the book: *Health does not need care!* None of you need any of us to keep your own health; it is a matter of personal responsibility! What you need us for is to provide *medical care* when disease affects you! In fact, let me restate that the tipping point of the downgrading of our system was precisely the shift from "Medical Care" to "Healthcare". The excuse that was used to dupe the entire country into this ideological change was that "Healthcare" implied a shift to *preventive care.* The supporters of such a change, proudly quoting Benjamin Franklin, bellowed from atop the mountain: *"An ounce of prevention is worth a pound of cure!"* However, let me introduce a smidge of reality; here is my own quote: *In the absolute, there is no such thing as preventive care!* Surprised? Skeptical? I understand that most of you would be. Nevertheless, some things are true whether you believe in them or not! Therefore, allow me the following explanation: Perhaps with the exception of vaccines, there is nothing we can do in medicine to prevent disease unless we are already treating something else. In other words, going to your primary doctor when you feel healthy for a regular check up, in and of itself cannot lead to the prevention of anything! I know that by now you must think I have completely lost it, but I assure you I can prove my point very easily. I dare you to pick any of the commonly held arguments for preventive care and examine it carefully. You will find that they are not all they are cut out to be. For example, performing mammograms does not prevent breast cancer; it just detects it early! Checking prostate specific antigen (PSA) does not prevent prostate cancer; it just detects it early! Sure one can argue that such initiatives prevent deaths. Really? I have more bad news; death cannot be prevented! Everyone is going to die sooner or later! The only thing we can aspire to do in medicine is to *prevent premature and unnecessary deaths!* This dovetails with the concept of temporarily prolonging life so long as it inherently has quality from the patient's perspective. Moreover, and along of what I said earlier, it is the *treatment* of hypertension, diabetes and abnormal cholesterol that impacts the prevention of stroke and heart attacks. So, the idea that disease prevention exists in a vacuum and that it represents the exclusive purview of primary care physicians is inaccurate and misleading. It is also the very concept that justified the creation and publicizing of Health Maintenance Organizations (HMOs) as a low cost and higher quality system of care. Look where that view has taken us!

To compound the problem, the acceptance of "Healthcare" *in lieu* of "Medical Care", with its implications in terms of preventive care, led to the inclusion of a whole variety of items that simply should have never been part of the mainstream practice of medicine. Let's take for example birth control. Whether we speak of prescribing oral contraceptives, performing vasectomies, or tubal ligations, the fact is that none of these tasks strictly speaking should be labeled as medical care, particularly when we consider that pregnancy is not a disease that needs prevention! However, by including birth control and other similar so-called preventive concerns into the scope of practice now called "Healthcare", we have unfocused the emphasis of our work, while adding a new dimension that was never meant to be. The cultural and economic implications of this change, which I insist must be undone, will become evident when we discuss the practical component of our solution. Suffice it to say, in my view, a return to the fundamental patient–physician relationship, accompanied by the restricted inclusion of those tasks that truly were meant to be part of medical care are *sine qua non* of any future solution. Harnessing the scope of practice and bringing it back to reality, while simultaneously shifting all extraneous factors to a non-essential level, should allow us better control of the delivery of medical care and all aspects related to it. It would be the first step in changing back to the original paradigm; the one that was originally meant to be!

After embracing the philosophical position I described above, we are ready to go ahead and dive into the discussion of the practical side of a solution. In my opinion, the only sensible approach to fixing the mess we currently call the healthcare system is the *Free Market*. Alas, nothing else will do! The advantage of this model is that it will afford us the ability to target all the players and dimensions of the system. The former include physicians, patients, insurance carriers, bureaucrats, allied health professionals, and legislators. The latter comprise accessibility, pricing, billing, insurance purchasing, drug approval, regulations, quality measurements, certification processes, and payment for services. Does this sound like a "comprehensive reform"? That certainly was not my intention! As a matter of fact, I think you should beware of any government legislation that includes the appellative of "comprehensive reform", for it is usually a bucket full of irrelevant statutes, rigid regulations, convoluted schedules, controlling mandates and hidden taxation. On the contrary, my vision is one of a solution that includes discrete components that can be examined, approved and executed independently, but yet can concurrently influence each other. You see, I think that the way we got to where we currently are is by a slow and gradual (i.e. step-by-step) downgrading of what once was an exceptional medical system. A little change here, a new regulation there, the force of the government behind it, and a progressive takeover of all aspects of our medical environment, either by federal institutions or their cronies (e.g. Blue Cross/Blue Shield). In fact, the downgrading of the American healthcare system has been nothing but a microcosm of the overall effect of the progressive political movement on our entire country over the last century, one characterized by increasing government control and regulations. Thus, it is only fair that we reverse the process in the same way: One step at a time! As I have shown in the previous chapters, every aspect of the current system is implicated in its downgrading and, therefore, every one of them must be brought to bear for a meaningful solution to actually be reached. To this end, I decided to present my proposed solution as a series of broad stroke recommendations for reform, each with its own set of intrinsic changes.

Less Government NOT More Government

It is only fitting, considering the information I have exposed throughout the book, that I tackle the government before any other of the system components, since it is the root cause of the mess in which we find ourselves. In considering the justification of this recommendation, I could not but remember a famous quote from Thomas Paine: *"It is the duty of every patriot to protect his country from its government!"* And so, it is eminently clear to me that the beginning of the downgrading process of the healthcare system was that moment when government began to meddle with it. I will cover the major financial repercussions of this fact in the context of insurance coverage and payment for services. Therefore, I will limit my present comments to the regulatory aspects of government intervention; those that allow it to exercise control over how care is to be delivered and, in the future, how much care and for whom! Indeed, the ACA (i.e. Obamacare) promises to introduce the largest degree of government control of healthcare in the history of our country. Thus, and without reservation, the first intrinsic change that must be considered is to repeal this law! Alas, unless the Republican candidate for President wins next November, AND has sufficient congressional back up to do so, we will continue down the road of medical serfdom until we become just like any other European nation!

However, repealing the ACA is not the end but just the beginning! Personally, I suggest that we walk backwards from the ACA, and take a critical look at each and every federal healthcare law passed since 1900 (especially those I have mentioned in the various chapters of this book), assessing its worth in the context of the following two queries: a) Is it redundant with any previous federal law (e.g. The Stark laws and the Federal Anti-kickback Statute)? And, b) Does it cover activities that the free market could steer more efficiently and effectively? Based upon these two criteria, it should be possible to slowly do away with every unnecessary regulatory constraint. Recently, the supporters of the ACA have demanded for anyone suggesting to have it repealed to produce a replacement alternative as a matter of demagoguery. The truth is that, as I mentioned above, a "comprehensive" law such as that is better replaced by multiple discrete initiatives that address laser-focused issues; only those not already covered by already existing legislation or better served by the invisible hand of the free market (as noted below). The immediate effect of this intrinsic change is the reduction of the *size* of the regulatory stranglehold of government on medical care, plus a *realignment* of many aspects of the latter with a more efficient way of operating within the nation's economy.

Along this line, the second intrinsic change I recommend is to audit the Department of Health and Human Services (DHHS), rename it the Department of Medical Affairs (DMA), and begin a process for reducing its scope of influence; restricting it to matters that truly belong in the realm of traditional *medical care* rather than encompassing numerous other politically correct issues that somehow seem to be appropriate solely in the context of *healthcare*. The immediate effect of this intrinsic change would be shrinkage of this cabinet post, with the resulting budgetary reductions. The latter could be subjected to additional yearly analyses as the rest of the present recommendations are implemented. The objective here is also to close any redundant programs and reduce wasteful spending. At the same time, removing the paternalistic and central-controlling influence of the government on medical care should induce a shift of priorities towards individual control, emphasizing once again the patient-physician functional unit described above. Part of this intrinsic change recommendation must also be extended to the government cronies; all the nonprofit organizations that have a voice ad influence pertinent to how medicine is practiced in our country. Any government endorsement of these entities should be critically assessed in the same light as the laws that have originated from their recommendations. Redundancy and duplication between them should be discouraged, as it contributes to sluggishness and exaggerated cost.

Medical Insurance NOT Healthcare Insurance

Let's present a small lesson in history prior to making our recommendations for intrinsic changes within this area of potential reform. The beginning of the 20th Century in our country saw a significant reluctance on the part of insurance companies to underwrite medical insurance. Primarily, this position obeyed the prevailing opinion that concepts such as "health" and "sickness" were vague terms that were prone to interpretation; as opposed for example to "death" (i.e. the subject of life insurance) which is very easy to define. In 1929, a group of 1,300 Dallas teachers formed a partnership with Baylor University Hospital based upon each of those making small monthly payments towards financing 21 days of inpatient care, should the need ever arise. This type of prepaid hospital care arrangement became popular during the depression, encouraged by the American Hospital Association (AHA) to the point that hospitals joined together under the name of *Blue Cross*. Ten years later, in 1939, physicians came together and formed their own prepaid plan for hospital-based physician services; and so, *Blue Shield* was born! It is important to note that this was called "accident and sickness insurance" not "health insurance", denoting the fact that they were meant to cover payment for catastrophic events that resulted in hospitalization. However, due to the influence of government regulations and the desire of politicians to be re-elected, the entire landscape has changed into what we have now. The result is that health insurance is nothing like any other type of insurance we currently buy! And that is why my intrinsic change recommendation in this section is to fundamentally convert it back into medical insurance.

In general, insurance constitutes a system by which people share the risk of an unanticipated loss, frequently accidental. It is not a group of people pooling money into a repository to eventually pay for expenses they expect to incur; it is certainly not a product they wish or plan to use! For example, when you buy car insurance, you do not want to have to use it, because that would mean you have had an accident! Furthermore, car insurance does not cover all routine services such as oil change, tire rotation, or even filling your tank with gas. If that were the case, can you imagine how expensive your premium payments would be? Ah! You just realized the fundamental difference between current health insurance and all other types of insurance. The fact that health insurance covers routine care (i.e. "health maintenance care") makes it equivalent to owning car insurance PLUS a very expensive maintenance plan! Hence, it is not surprising that the cost of health insurance continues to soar: It is covering items above and beyond medical care! Unless this paradigm is reversed, there is no hope to control the exorbitant growth of its cost.

Along this line, if we embrace the philosophical principle of replacing "healthcare" with the traditional "medical care", and tailor insurance within the constraints of this concept, we would arrive at a balanced situation whereby the insurance would only pay for major medical issues, while routine care would be the responsibility of the patient. The immediate effects of this intrinsic change would include: a) Reduction of insurance premiums; b) Realistic view of medical care prices by the patient who has to be able to afford routine care services; and c) Exclusion of services that are not strictly speaking "medical" (e.g. any form of contraception) from coverage. Now, I am sure this is going to meet with significant resistance but the alternative is to continue down a path that will result in further expansion of the cost of care, with little hope for avoiding the rationing imposed by the government.

Additionally, applying a free market model to medical insurance (we would no longer call it health insurance) would include removing all mandates for coverage and, in turn, allowing the purchasing of medical insurance across state lines. Why? Because, at present, courtesy of our stellar elected officials, every single state has a different number and set of health insurance coverage mandates! How different are they? Vastly! For example, Rhode Island has 69 mandates, Idaho only has 13 and my state, Alabama, has a mere 19! By leveling the field through mandates removal, it becomes feasible for medical insurance carriers to compete across states. This degree of competition should have a beneficial effect on prices. Moreover, for those who wish to have their routine care (including contraception if you will) covered, supplementary insurance may then be purchased for additional fees, or they resort to *Medical Savings Accounts (MSA)* as noted below. Also, under this more logical system, individuals with higher risk would necessarily have to pay somewhat higher premiums, creating an incentive for responsibility and accountability about one's own health status. Yes, this is going to cost individuals some money. However, we are already contributing large amounts of our income to the payment of very expensive employer-based insurance premiums. Besides, if we also include tax reform legislation allowing individuals to pay for any type of medical insurance using pre-tax dollars, we would significantly soften the financial burden of this paradigm. In this context, such a degree of freedom would negate the need for any additional legislation pertinent to pre-existing conditions, or to prevent employers from dropping employees from their plans.

Needless to say, the Centers for Medicare and Medicaid Services (CMS) would have to be remodeled to fit within the new free market paradigm. This would have to include some form of privatization, the use of special MSAs, and the patient having more control of how his federally allocated dollars are spent, rather being told by CMS what they are covered for or not. Although the supporters of a progressive agenda with continued mismanagement of CMS funds would make accusations about *"trying to end Medicare as we know it!"* the truth is that *"as we know it"* Medicare is inexorably gravitating towards financial extinction. In the next section I will cover the backbone of the entire new system I recommend: *Price-based interactions!*

Prize-Based Exchanges NOT Centralized Reimbursement

An essential aspect of the free market is the role played by prices in guiding the decisions of consumers. Prices include information about supply and demand, and give individuals a sense of their acquisitive power at a moment in time. Needless to say, in the present healthcare system, prices do not mean anything since they are artificially fixed by the government and its cronies (Chapter 7). That means that the average patient does not have a realistic view of the cost and prices of the medical transactions pertinent to his own health. Thus, the intrinsic change recommended in this section is an open and transparent use of a free pricing system; physicians and hospitals would have the freedom to set their prices, while patients would have the freedom to choose how their medical dollars are spent. They would be able to compare and contrast, research the best deal, and investigate issues of quality. The perfect vehicle for the implementation of this intrinsic change, from the perspective of patients, is that of MSAs. In our model described in the previous section, I emphasized how patients would be responsible for payment of certain services that are not strictly medical care (e.g. screening tests); those that are part of routine care. Even though the current rhetoric is that a large percentage of our population is underinsured when it comes to their medical care, the truth is that there are many who are spending a significant amount of money in insurance premiums to cover services they could pay out-of-pocket at a lesser rate. In other words, to give an insurance company $2 to cover a service that costs only $1, does not make any sense whatsoever! Therefore, it is important for patients to recognize that it is possible to assume some of the financial responsibility of paying for medical care, particularly the less expensive routine services, by virtue of having savings accounts that are dedicated for this purpose. In general, MSAs are part of plans with relatively high deductibles, paid by the individual either out-of-pocket or from the MSA itself. The insurance company would then cover all expenses after the deductible has been met. Both the employer and the employee can add money to the MSA, but the premise is that by setting this money aside, the individual has more control of how these dollars are spent. In combination with a price-based system, this model would empower patients in much better ways than the current system does. In addition, any money that is not spent rolls over and continues to grow tax-free. Later, at age 65, the individual has access to these funds even though they are subject to regular income taxes. Unfortunately, the existing laws significantly restrict how

MSAs are managed and, therefore, legislative changes would be required in order for MSAs to be more flexible than they currently are. More specifically, the creation of MSAs similar to those currently operating in South Africa seems like a very attractive alternative to the current state of affairs. A potential criticism of this degree of freedom and empowerment of patients is that they could make incorrect financial decisions about medical services, spending more money than necessary. However, every single study looking at this issue over the last thirty years has almost invariably shown the opposite. When patients are managing their own money, and have access to realistic prices, the results in general have included a reduction in unnecessary expenditures. On the supply side, when providers are faced with patients who spend their medical dollars more prudently, they are steered into price transparency and price competition. The latter, almost unequivocally results in quality competition (see below).

Interestingly, a similar approach would even work for Medicare and Medicaid. As a matter of fact, having these patients control their medical expenditures via special MSAs would create a more realistic environment, less fraught with fraud and abuse because every single patient would be his own watchdog! In turn, this may allow the newly created DMA to reduce its fraud and abuse investigation budget! Ain't that a peach?

Physicians NOT Health Care Providers

The principal role of the physician in the delivery of medical care, as acknowledged in the philosophical component described above is of paramount importance. Clearly, physicians must step up to the plate but, should they do so, their education and expertise must be recognized. The redesign of the process must begin by stopping all reform activities in medical education, and emphasizing a return to the fundamental principles that made our country a medically exceptional one. Emphasis in a strong basic science foundation, a shift from data memorization to critical thinking, and an expansion of the concept of Evidence Based Medicine (EBM) to the format originally intended (Figure 2-5), are necessarily part of this intrinsic change recommendation. So would be the recognition of physician individuality in practice, the fact that guidelines are not dogma, and that rules must be constantly broken by the innovation that engenders new rules.

Once this transformation back to the basis takes place, particularly after the arduous road required for becoming a practicing physician, there has to be a commensurate alignment of authority. No more second guessing; no more forms to fill; no more shenanigans relative to the physician's authority in the care of the patients who have placed their trust in him! Allow physicians to occupy their rightful place as the leaders of the clinical team, and subordinate the operations of the system to the realization of the physician-patient relationship in its full form. Conversely, have little latitude towards physicians who breach the confidence placed on them by the system: Zero tolerance! Have the incompetent, suboptimal, negligent, and dishonest physicians removed and excised from the system without hesitation! This set of changes alone should guarantee an improvement in quality of care, without the need for surveys, paperwork or bureaucracy. Along these lines, it should be possible to demand transparency at all levels, without witch-hunts or presumption of guilt, thereby freeing the entrepreneurial spirit of physicians, and contributing to their contribution to the free market of medical care.

Patients NOT Entitled Citizens

In the same manner as I have recommended changing the role of the physician back to his original place in the basic construct of medical care, a similar change must occur to his partner, the patient. This is probably one of the most difficult changes to effect, since the current issues derive from widespread cultural changes that cannot be easily corrected. However, instilling the financial and economic freedom described, and providing the patient with increased control over his own medical destiny, are likely to create the perfect starting point.

Introducing a set of responsibilities that would match those rights patients seem to be so eager to exercise can easily follow this. The main concept of the present intrinsic change recommendation is that of creating a culture of patient accountability, particularly as the product of assigning him an equal (not identical) role to that of his physician at the core of the system. It is only by following this path that we can only empower individuals, changing their expectations and facilitating how they view life in general, and particularly as it relates to the treatment of medical conditions. The expectation here is also that such a change in attitude would translate in increased happiness, perhaps the most important determining factor for the maintenance of health. Additional benefits of a cultural change of the patient population is also bound to have phenomenal implications with respect to my practice issues, as well as a more clear understanding of pertinent legislative issues relative to medical care. Finally, having patients "do their part" across the medical care continuum is also of potential benefit in improving quality and safety.

Outcomes NOT Processes

As I already mentioned, striving for quality and a passion for excellence are worthy attributes for a system transformation in the right direction. However, the intrinsic change recommendation relevant to this topic is that of focusing on results and not on processes. Individuals should have the freedom to pursue any course of action, however different, so long as their results leave no room for doubt about excellence in care. In general, assessment of these outcomes should not be in the hands of the government or its surrogates.

A significant shift from the current methodology of having all forms filled, all checkboxes checked, and all steps covered irrespective of the outcome of the patient is perhaps one of the most important changes we can make to the current system. As I noted earlier, the inordinate focus on processes obviates the fact that none of them guarantees excellence in outcome. Furthermore, it allows for mediocrity to be part of the system by means of covering for providers incapable of operating without a set of instructions. It also assumes that every patient is exactly identical to the next, not allowing for the provision of care tailored to the specific individual.

More Education NOT More Regulation

Another aspect of our current regulations that has to be reduced is that of licensing and regulations. The elimination of the medieval guild system was an early necessary step in the rise of freedom in the western hemisphere. Finally, men could pursue any occupation of their choice without requiring permission from the government or its surrogate agencies. At present, however, the licensing processes for physicians, nurses and other health professions have revitalized control and restriction of trade by the apposite groups. Much like the medieval guilds, licensed professionals with economic interest in the control of their profession constitute their respective licensing and certifying boards. These boards control entrance into the profession, and exercise continued control throughout the career of every practitioner. It is almost as if it is never enough! One is never finished with proving himself in the eyes of these "authoritative" organizations.

The intrinsic change recommendation in this section is that of placing an emphasis in real education rather than in a chain of meaningless certifications, licenses and regulations that accomplish nothing but to restrict the physician's ability to pursue his aspirations. Remember that the longstanding justification for all of these certificates and licenses, as well as the regulations that frame them, is that of *"assuring quality"*. However, I would like to share one last anecdote that proves that, if we embrace a culture that rewards excellence and cultivates integrity, we have little to worry, and so do our patients.

Although earlier in the book I indicated that I thought the most important quality of a physician was the ability to integrate information, I recently posed this question to a very dear friend and colleague of mine; a neurosurgeon with over twenty years of experience. As it happens, he is also a mathematician, has a business degree (we were classmates at the University of Tennessee), and is probably just about the smartest person I know. His answer, which at this time I find incredibly relevant was: *Moral Compass!* I certainly cannot argue the importance of this attribute, particularly because I find it indispensable as we recommend a system-wide reduction of regulations, laws, and restrictions that exist because the government insists to "look out for us". The truth is that if we concentrate our efforts in carefully choosing the individuals that are going to participate in our system of medical care as providers, we are unlikely to need arbitrary constraints; to quote Benjamin Disraeli, *"When men are pure, laws are useless; when men are corrupt, laws are broken."*

Outlook

In summary, there is hope for our medical system, even if slim. It would not be easy to fix but the possible solution I propose includes the philosophical necessity to return to the fundamental core values of embracing: a) The Basic Physician-Patient Relationship, and b) The Medical Care Paradigm. Such a conceptual transformation would have to be followed by a practical strategy based on a return to the free market. Rather than follow the common political path of "comprehensive reform", loaded with a variety of pitfalls and shortcomings, a series of discrete and laser-focused changes seem to be much more reasonable. The path I propose should lead to changes characterized by less government involvement, realistic medical insurance, a price-based economic model, emphasis on true physician leadership, decreased medical entitlements, enhanced role of education, and a focus on outcomes as a quality metric.

This all sounds almost impossible to achieve, doesn't it? Well, as I have often said, *"It is always darkest... ...before it turns pitch black!"* and, in my opinion, we have not yet hit rock bottom. In fact, I suspect our system is bound to see further downgrading before we can intervene to fix it. Perhaps it will be necessary for it to deteriorate to the point of imminent collapse before anyone is willing to make hard choices. Moreover, after reading all these pages, the naysayers may criticize my suggestions, labeling them as unrealistic and illusory. They may be right… …or maybe not! There may indeed be other ways to repair our system. As for myself, all I can say is that *I may be willing to compromise in strategy but never in principles!*

A Final Thought...

"It is not the critic who counts, not the man who points out how the strong man stumbled, or where the doer of deeds could have done better. The credit belongs to the man who is actually in the arena; whose face is marred by the dust and sweat and blood; who strives valiantly; who errs and comes short again and again; who knows the great enthusiasms, the great devotions and spends himself in a worthy course; who at best, knows in the end the triumph of high achievement, and who, at worst, if he fails, at least fails while daring greatly; so that his place shall never be with those cold and timid souls who know neither victory or defeat."

Theodore Roosevelt
26th President of the United States
(1858 - 1919)

SELECTED READING

(PhRMA), Pharmaceutical Research and Manufacturers of America. 2009. Code on Interactions with Healthcare

Professionals. http://www.pharma.com: Pharmaceutical Research and Manufacturers of America (PhRMA).

America, Committee on Quality of Health Care in, and Institute of Medicine. 2000. *To Err Is Human: Building a Safer Health System.* Edited by Linda T. Kohn, Janet M. Corrigan and Molla S. Donaldson: The National Academies Press.

———. 2001. *Crossing the Quality Chasm: A New Health System for the 21st Century*: The National Academies Press.

Andrews, L. B., C. Stocking, T. Krizek, L. Gottlieb, C. Krizek, T. Vargish, and M. Siegler. 1997. "An alternative strategy for studying adverse events in medical care." *Lancet* no. 349 (9048):309-13. doi: 10.1016/S0140-6736(96)08268-2.

Anonymous. 2009. *In Sickness and in Health: The History of Health Insurance.* Random History 2009 [cited March 31, 2009 2009]. Available from http://www.randomhistory.com/2009/03/31_health-nsurance.html.

Belknap, S. M. 2010. "ACP Journal Club. Review: Rapid-response teams do not reduce mortality in hospital patients." *Ann Intern Med* no. 152 (12):JC6-3. doi: 10.1059/0003-4819-152-12-201006150-02003.

Bhatt, S. 1995. "Academic medicine undergoes revolution." *The Chronile.*

Brennan, T. A., L. L. Leape, N. M. Laird, L. Hebert, A. R. Localio, A. G. Lawthers, J. P. Newhouse, P. C. Weiler, and H. H. Hiatt. 1991. "Incidence of adverse events and negligence in hospitalized patients. Results of the Harvard Medical Practice Study I." *N Engl J Med* no. 324 (6):370-6. doi: 10.1056/NEJM199102073240604.

Brott, T. G., E. C. Haley, Jr., D. E. Levy, W. Barsan, J. Broderick, G. L. Sheppard, J. Spilker, G. L. Kongable, S. Massey, R. Reed, and et al. 1992. "Urgent therapy for stroke. Part I. Pilot study of tissue plasminogen activator administered within 90 minutes." *Stroke* no. 23 (5):632-40.

Brown, T. 2012. "Hospitals Aren't Hotels." *The New York Times*, March 14, 2012.

Buist, M. D., G. E. Moore, S. A. Bernard, B. P. Waxman, J. N. Anderson, and T. V. Nguyen. 2002. "Effects of a medical emergency team on reduction of incidence of and mortality from unexpected cardiac arrests in hospital: preliminary study." *BMJ* no. 324 (7334):387-90.

Caplan, L. R. 2002. "Is the promise of randomized control trials ("evidence-based medicine") overstated?" *Curr Neurol Neurosci Rep* no. 2 (1):1-8.

Care, Committee on the Future of Emergency, and in the United States Health System. 2007. *Hospital-Based Emergency Care: At the Breaking*

Point, Futures of Emerfency Care. Washington, DC: The National Academies Press.

Charrois, T. L., M. Zolezzi, S. L. Koshman, G. Pearson, M. Makowsky, T. Durec, and R. T. Tsuyuki. 2012. "A systematic review of the evidence for pharmacist care of patients with dyslipidemia." *Pharmacotherapy* no. 32 (3):222-33. doi: 10.1002/j.1875-9114.2012.01022.x.

Chassin, M. R., J. M. Loeb, S. P. Schmaltz, and R. M. Wachter. 2010. "Accountability measures--using measurement to promote quality improvement." *N Engl J Med* no. 363 (7):683-8. doi: 10.1056/NEJMsb1002320.

Committee on Advancing Pain Research, Care, and Education, and Board on Health Sciences Policy. 2011. *Relieving Pain in America: A Blueprint for Transforming*

Prevention, Care, Education, and Research. Washington, DC: The National Academies Press.

Cuff, PA, and NA Vanselow. 2004. *Enhancing the Behavioral and Social Science*

Content of Medical School Curricula. Washington, DC: National Academies Press.

Daffurn, K., A. Lee, K. M. Hillman, G. F. Bishop, and A. Bauman. 1994. "Do nurses know when to summon emergency assistance?" *Intensive Crit Care Nurs* no. 10 (2):115-20.

DeVita, M. A., and R. Bellomo. 2007. "The case of rapid response systems: are randomized clinical trials the right methodology to evaluate systems of care?" *Crit Care Med* no. 35 (5):1413-4. doi: 10.1097/01.CCM.0000262729.63882.57.

Dewalt, D. A., N. D. Berkman, S. Sheridan, K. N. Lohr, and M. P. Pignone. 2004. "Literacy and health outcomes: a systematic review of the literature." *J Gen Intern Med* no. 19 (12):1228-39. doi: 10.1111/j.1525-1497.2004.40153.x.

Flexner, A. 2002. "Medical education in the United States and Canada. From the Carnegie Foundation for the Advancement of Teaching, Bulletin Number Four, 1910." *Bull World Health Organ* no. 80 (7):594-602.

Galhotra, S., M. A. DeVita, R. L. Simmons, and M. A. Dew. 2007. "Mature rapid response system and potentially avoidable cardiopulmonary arrests in hospital." *Qual Saf Health Care* no. 16 (4):260-5. doi: 10.1136/qshc.2007.022210.

Gawande, A. A., M. J. Zinner, D. M. Studdert, and T. A. Brennan. 2003. "Analysis of errors reported by surgeons at three teaching hospitals." *Surgery* no. 133 (6):614-21. doi: 10.1067/msy.2003.169.

Graham, R, M Mancher, DM Wolman, S Greenfield, and E Steinberg. 2011. *Clinical Practice Guidelines we can Trust.* Washington, DC: The National Academies Press.

Greiner, AC, and E Knebel. 2003. *Health Professions Education: A Bridge to Quality*. Washington, DC: The National Academies Press.

Haley, E. C., Jr., D. E. Levy, T. G. Brott, G. L. Sheppard, M. C. Wong, G. L. Kongable, J. C. Torner, and J. R. Marler. 1992. "Urgent therapy for stroke. Part II. Pilot study of tissue plasminogen activator administered 91-180 minutes from onset." *Stroke* no. 23 (5):641-5.

Healy, D. 2006. "The latest mania: selling bipolar disorder." *PLoS Med* no. 3 (4):e185. doi: 10.1371/journal.pmed.0030185.

Hillman, K., J. Chen, M. Cretikos, R. Bellomo, D. Brown, G. Doig, S. Finfer, and A. Flabouris. 2005. "Introduction of the medical emergency team (MET) system: a cluster-randomised controlled trial." *Lancet* no. 365 (9477):2091-7. doi: 10.1016/S0140-6736(05)66733-5.

Hillman, K., M. DeVita, R. Bellomo, and J. Chen. 2010. "Meta-analysis for rapid response teams." *Arch Intern Med* no. 170 (11):996-7; author reply 997. doi: 10.1001/archinternmed.2010.178.

Hulkower, R. 2010. "The History of the Hippocratic Oath: Outdated, Inauthentic, and Yet Still Relevant." *EJBM*:41-44.

Jacobs, L. 2009. "Interview with Lawrence Weed, MD- The Father of the Problem-Oriented Medical Record Looks Ahead." *Perm J* no. 13 (3):84-9.

Jagsi, R., J. Shapiro, and D. F. Weinstein. 2005. "Perceived impact of resident work hour limitations on medical student clerkships: a survey study." *Acad Med* no. 80 (8):752-7.

Jagsi, R., J. Shapiro, J. S. Weissman, D. J. Dorer, and D. F. Weinstein. 2006. "The educational impact of ACGME limits on resident and fellow duty hours: a pre-post survey study." *Acad Med* no. 81 (12):1059-68. doi: 10.1097/01.ACM.0000246685.96372.5e.

Johnson, Committee on the Robert Wood, Foundation Initiative on the Future of Nursing, and at the Institute of Medicine. 2010. *A Summary of the February 2010 Forum on the Future of Nursing: Education*. Washington, DC: The National Academies Press.

Jones, D. A., M. A. DeVita, and R. Bellomo. 2011. "Rapid-response teams." *N Engl J Med* no. 365 (2):139-46. doi: 10.1056/NEJMra0910926.

Kellermann, A. L. 2006. "Crisis in the emergency department." *N Engl J Med* no. 355 (13):1300-3. doi: 10.1056/NEJMp068194.

Kripalani, S., and B. D. Weiss. 2006. "Teaching about health literacy and clear communication." *J Gen Intern Med* no. 21 (8):888-90. doi: 10.1111/j.1525-1497.2006.00543.x.

Kusserow, RP. 1989. FINANCIAL ARRANGEMENTS BETWEEN PHYSICIANS AND HEALTH CARE BUSINESSES. edited by Office of Analysis and INspections: Office of Inspector General.

Kwaan, M. R., D. M. Studdert, M. J. Zinner, and A. A. Gawande. 2006. "Incidence, patterns, and prevention of wrong-site surgery." *Arch Surg* no. 141 (4):353-7; discussion 357-8. doi: 10.1001/archsurg.141.4.353.

Landrigan, C. P., S. W. Lockley, and C. A. Czeisler. 2005. "Effect of intern's consecutive work hours on safety, medical education and professionalism." *Crit Care* no. 9 (5):528-30; author reply 528-30. doi: 10.1186/cc3730.

Landrigan, C. P., J. M. Rothschild, J. W. Cronin, R. Kaushal, E. Burdick, J. T. Katz, C. M. Lilly, P. H. Stone, S. W. Lockley, D. W. Bates, and C. A. Czeisler. 2004. "Effect of reducing interns' work hours on serious medical errors in intensive care units." *N Engl J Med* no. 351 (18):1838-48. doi: 10.1056/NEJMoa041406.

Leape, L. L., T. A. Brennan, N. Laird, A. G. Lawthers, A. R. Localio, B. A. Barnes, L. Hebert, J. P. Newhouse, P. C. Weiler, and H. Hiatt. 1991. "The nature of adverse events in hospitalized patients. Results of the Harvard Medical Practice Study II." *N Engl J Med* no. 324 (6):377-84. doi: 10.1056/NEJM199102073240605.

Lee, A., G. Bishop, K. M. Hillman, and K. Daffurn. 1995. "The Medical Emergency Team." *Anaesth Intensive Care* no. 23 (2):183-6.

Levinson, DR. 2008. ADVERSE EVENTS IN HOSPITALS: OVERVIEW OF KEY ISSUES. edited by Office of the INspectore General. Washington, DC: Department of Health and Human Service.

McClellan, MB, JM McGinnis, EG Nabel, and LM Olsen. 2008. "Evidence-Based Medicine and the Changing Nature of Healthcare: Meeting Summary (IOM Roundtable on Evidence-Based Medicine)." In *2007 IOM Annual Meeting Series*. Washington, DC: The National Academy Press.

McClure, M. L. 2005. "Magnet hospitals: insights and issues." *Nurs Adm Q* no. 29 (3):198-201.

Mitchell, J. M., and E. Scott. 1992. "Physician ownership of physical therapy services. Effects on charges, utilization, profits, and service characteristics." *JAMA* no. 268 (15):2055-9.

Moynihan, R. 2006. "Scientists find new disease: motivational deficiency disorder." *BMJ* no. 332:745.

Mularski, R. A., F. White-Chu, D. Overbay, L. Miller, S. M. Asch, and L. Ganzini. 2006. "Measuring pain as the 5th vital sign does not improve quality of pain management." *J Gen Intern Med* no. 21 (6):607-12. doi: 10.1111/j.1525-1497.2006.00415.x.

Nisen, L. 2011. "Pharmacist prescribing: What are the next steps?" *Am J Health-Syst Pharm* (68):2357-61.

O'Sulivan, J. 2007. Medicare: Physician Self Referral ("Stark I and II"). edited by Congress Research Service. Report to Congress.

Pearson, J. T., and W. N. Pitkethly. 1969. "The pharmacist in industry." *Chem Br* no. 5 (8):360-2.

Pearson, K. 1982. "The pharmacist and adverse drug reaction reporting." *Hosp Pharm* no. 17 (8):421-2, 427-30.

Poses, R. M. 1997. "Estimation of adverse events in medical care." *Lancet* no. 349 (9056):959. doi: 10.1016/S0140-6736(05)62744-4.

Relman, A. S. 1980. "The new medical-industrial complex." *N Engl J Med* no. 303 (17):963-70. doi: 10.1056/NEJM198010233031703.

Rogers, S. O., Jr., A. A. Gawande, M. Kwaan, A. L. Puopolo, C. Yoon, T. A. Brennan, and D. M. Studdert. 2006. "Analysis of surgical errors in closed malpractice claims at 4 liability insurers." *Surgery* no. 140 (1):25-33. doi: 10.1016/j.surg.2006.01.008.

Shikles, JL. 1993. Physicians Who Invest in Imaging Centers Refer More Patients for More Costly Services. In *Ways and Means*, edited by Health Financing and Policy Issues: United States General Accounting Office.

Simon, S. K., K. Phillips, S. Badalamenti, J. Ohlert, and J. Krumberger. 1997. "Current practices regarding visitation policies in critical care units." *Am J Crit Care* no. 6 (3):210-7.

Skochelak, S. E. 2010. "A decade of reports calling for change in medical education: what do they say?" *Acad Med* no. 85 (9 Suppl):S26-33. doi: 10.1097/ACM.0b013e3181f1323f.

Smith, G. C., and J. P. Pell. 2003. "Parachute use to prevent death and major trauma related to gravitational challenge: systematic review of randomised controlled trials." *BMJ* no. 327 (7429):1459-61. doi: 10.1136/bmj.327.7429.1459.

Sobel, R. 2007. "The HIPAA paradox: the privacy rule that's not." *The Hastings Center Report* no. 37 (4):40-51.

Studdert, D. M., M. M. Mello, and T. A. Brennan. 2004. "Medical malpractice." *N Engl J Med* no. 350 (3):283-92. doi: 10.1056/NEJMhpr035470.

Studdert, D. M., M. M. Mello, A. A. Gawande, T. K. Gandhi, A. Kachalia, C. Yoon, A. L. Puopolo, and T. A. Brennan. 2006. "Claims, errors, and compensation payments in medical malpractice litigation." *N Engl J Med* no. 354 (19):2024-33. doi: 10.1056/NEJMsa054479.

Studdert, D. M., E. J. Thomas, H. R. Burstin, B. I. Zbar, E. J. Orav, and T. A. Brennan. 2000. "Negligent care and malpractice claiming behavior in Utah and Colorado." *Med Care* no. 38 (3):250-60.

Committee on the Robert Wood Johnson Foundation Initiative on Future of Nursing. 2011. *The Future of Nursing: Leading Change, Advancing Health*. Edited by The Institute of Medicine. Washington, DC: The National Academies Press.

Thomas, E. J., D. M. Studdert, H. R. Burstin, E. J. Orav, T. Zeena, E. J. Williams, K. M. Howard, P. C. Weiler, and T. A. Brennan. 2000. "Incidence and types of adverse events and negligent care in Utah and Colorado." *Med Care* no. 38 (3):261-71.

Triggle, D. J. 2007. "Treating desires not diseases: a pill for every ill and an ill for every pill?" *Drug Discov Today* no. 12 (3-4):161-6. doi: 10.1016/j.drudis.2006.12.001.

Tufo, H. M., R. E. Bouchard, A. S. Rubin, J. C. Twitchell, H. C. VanBuren, L. B. Weed, and M. Rothwell. 1977. "Problem-oriented approach to practice. I. Economic impact." *JAMA* no. 238 (5):414-7.

VanSuch, M., J. M. Naessens, R. J. Stroebel, J. M. Huddleston, and A. R. Williams. 2006. "Effect of discharge instructions on readmission of hospitalised patients with heart failure: do all of the Joint Commission on Accreditation of Healthcare Organizations heart failure core measures reflect better care?" *Qual Saf Health Care* no. 15 (6):414-7. doi: 10.1136/qshc.2005.017640.

Weed, L. 1975. "The problem-oriented record-its organizing principles and its structure." *League Exch* (103):3-6.

Weed, L. L. 1971. "The problem oriented record as a basic tool in medical education, patient care and clinical research." *Ann Clin Res* no. 3 (3):131-4.

Weed, L. L., and N. J. Zimny. 1989. "The problem-oriented system, problem-knowledge coupling, and clinical decision making." *Phys Ther* no. 69 (7):565-8.

Winters, B. D., J. C. Pham, E. A. Hunt, E. Guallar, S. Berenholtz, and P. J. Pronovost. 2007. "Rapid response systems: a systematic review." *Crit Care Med* no. 35 (5):1238-43. doi: 10.1097/01.CCM.0000262388.85669.68.

Winters, B. D., J. Pham, and P. J. Pronovost. 2006. "Rapid response teams--walk, don't run." *JAMA* no. 296 (13):1645-7. doi: 10.1001/jama.296.13.1645.

Yamada, C., J. A. Johnson, P. Robertson, G. Pearson, and R. T. Tsuyuki. 2005. "Long-term impact of a community pharmacist intervention on cholesterol levels in patients at high risk for cardiovascular events: extended follow-up of the second study of cardiovascular risk intervention by pharmacists (SCRIP-plus)." *Pharmacotherapy* no. 25 (1):110-5. doi: 10.1592/phco.25.1.110.55619.

www.ingramcontent.com/pod-product-compliance
Lightning Source LLC
Chambersburg PA
CBHW051438170526
45166CB00001B/29
9781475069822